I0025821

THE STRESS-ILLNESS CONNECTION

A SIMPLE GUIDE TO UNDERSTANDING THE PHYSICAL AND EMOTIONAL CAUSES OF DISEASE

Easy to Read
Fully Backed by Science

Amy Lewis

The Stress-Illness Connection © Amy Lewis 2025

ISBN: 978-1-923476-57-8 (paperback)

All rights reserved. No part of this publication may be reproduced, stored in a retrieval system, or transmitted in any form or by any means electronic, mechanical, photocopying, recording, or otherwise, without the prior written permission of the author.

NATIONAL
LIBRARY
OF AUSTRALIA

A catalogue record for this
book is available from the
National Library of Australia

To all of humanity who are suffering

Contents

Introduction

The world we live in today is very different from life on Earth many centuries ago. Life is busy; people work full-time and try to balance that with family life. The world has just suffered a pandemic and there is a rise in the cost of living, forcing people to lose their homes or rentals. There are multiple wars in several countries, and terrorism has caused a state of fear on the planet. Drug and alcohol addiction are prevalent. Narcissistic personalities on a varying spectrum are on the rise, and this can negatively impact relationships, leading to situations of domestic violence and child abuse. There are so many ultra-processed food options at the supermarket and it's hard not to be tempted. These include lollies, chips, cookies, and packaged food with Monosodium Glutamate (MSG) and many numbers, preservatives, colourings, and additives. Fruit, vegetables, and grains are not pesticide-free, unless you buy certified organic. When we get sick, our doctors might order many scans such as X-rays, Computed Tomography (CT), and Positron Emission Tomography (PET) scans, and nuclear medicine scans, which expose us to ionising radiation. Viruses are theorised to be an underlying cause of cancer. All these factors place stress on our mind, body, and soul.

This book is a simple guide to understanding what stress is in all its forms and how stress can provoke the manifestation of dis-ease/ illness within the body. It's important for humanity to be aware of this stress-illness connection to empower us to make choices that promote health and healing, daily.

Chapter 1

Illness in the 21st Century

Either you or someone you know might be suffering from a disease. A disease or dis-ease is defined as a sickness or instance of sickness or a condition in which the function and often the structure of the body or part of the body is disturbed or impaired.[1] This can include impaired mental function. The sickness may have characteristic signs and symptoms and there may be something that has caused it to occur.[2]

Diseases are either an infectious disease (communicable) that can be transferred from person to person, such as the flu, or a disease that is not infectious (non-communicable), meaning a disease that is not spread from person to person, such as cancer, heart disease, kidney disease, or diabetes.[3] Both infectious and non-infectious diseases can be acute or chronic in nature (see Figure 1.1). An acute disease has a sudden appearance of signs and symptoms and lasts only a short time, for example, infections or injuries such as influenza A or a broken bone or an ankle sprain.[4] A chronic disease or condition lasts a long time or a lifetime, such as cancer, asthma, heart disease, kidney disease, or diabetes.[5]

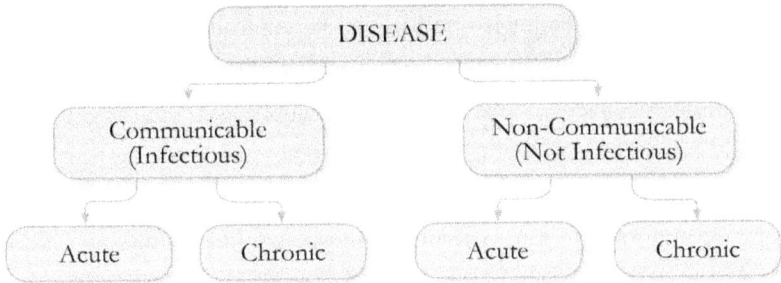

```
                          DISEASE

        Communicable                    Non-Communicable
        (Infectious)                    (Not Infectious)

    Acute         Chronic             Acute          Chronic
```

Figure 1.1

Often, people suffer from more than one chronic disease and their state of health becomes complex.[6] People might suffer from one chronic disease, and others develop because of the original disease. An example of this is high blood pressure and the consequent development of cardiovascular disease.[7] Chronic diseases such as cancer and cardiovascular disease develop over time.[8] Some chronic diseases often lead to disability and frailty in later life[9]. Chronic diseases, thus, have been called the pandemic of the 21st century, both in developing and developed countries.[10]

A risk factor is a characteristic or a hazard that can predispose a person to getting an acute or chronic disease.[11] There are two types of risk factors: modifiable and non-modifiable (see Figure 1.2).

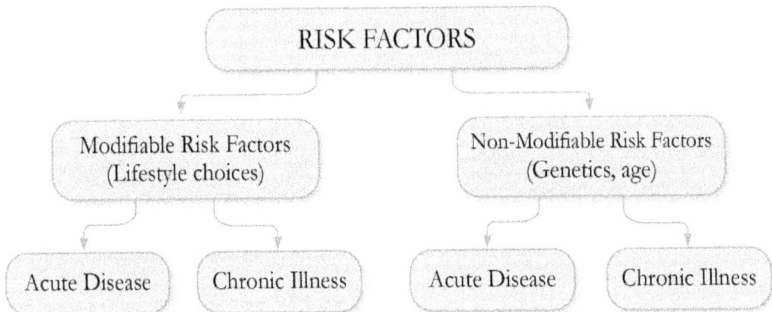

```
                        RISK FACTORS

     Modifiable Risk Factors              Non-Modifiable Risk Factors
     (Lifestyle choices)                  (Genetics, age)

   Acute Disease   Chronic Illness      Acute Disease    Chronic Illness
```

Figure 1.2

A modifiable risk factor is one that can be controlled or changed and can cause stress on a person's body, such as lifestyle choices. A non-modifiable risk factor is one that cannot be controlled, such as genetics. Stress in all its forms, being physical, mental, emotional and spiritual, can and does affect the physical body and both acute and chronic disease may result[12]. Stress-related illnesses are increasing, more than at any other time in history.[13] Firstly, let us explore what stress is.

Chapter 2

What is Stress?

Definition of Stress

The World Health Organisation defines stress as "a state of worry or mental tension caused by a difficult situation."[14] Hans Selye, an Austrian-born Hungarian scientist, was nominated for the Nobel Prize for discovering, in 1936, the condition of "stress."[15] Selye stated that stress can be defined as "the non-specific response of the body to any demand for change" and "is essentially the state of wear and tear caused by life" and, moreover, that "Stress is the spice of life."[16] More about the stress response that Selye discovered will be discussed in Chapter 3. Scientifically, stress is essentially a state of threatened homeodynamic (normal state) balance by a wide range of internal or external, real or perceived challenges or stimuli.[17] These challenges or stimuli that cause stress are called a "stressor" and can be further broken down into psychological and physical stressors that can affect both physical and/or mental health. Firstly, let's look at some psychological stressors.

Psychological Stressors

A psychological stressor is something that triggers an emotional stress response.[18] Some psychological stressors are:

- Work
- Family
- Relationships

- Miscellaneous life events
- Employment
- Academic
- Mental health disorders

The following list of life events or experiences, and their corresponding scores on the right, is called The Social Readjustment Rating Scale (SRRS). It is a scoring system that allows for insight into the risk of developing an illness after one or more stressful life events. [19] How these psychological stressors cause illness will be discussed in Chapter 3.

The list is ranked from the highest stress experiences to the lowest, as described by Leah Hechtman in her book *Clinical Naturopathic Medicine* (2012).[20]

How to Use the SRRS:

Add up the scores (on the right) of all the life events you have experienced in the past year.

If your score is greater than 200, you are at a higher risk of illness.

If your score is 150-200, you are at moderate risk of illness (30% reduced from the above risk).

If your score is less than 150, you are at minimal risk of illness.

This list applies to adults:

1. Death of a spouse..100
2. Divorce...73
3. Marital separation..65
4. Imprisonment...63
5. Death of a close family member..63
6. Personal injury or illness...53
7. Marriage...50
8. Fired/dismissal from work..47
9. Marital reconciliation...45
10. Retirement..45
11. Change in health of family member..44
12. Pregnancy...40
13. Sexual difficulties...39
14. Gain of a new family member...39
15. Business adjustment...39
16. Change in financial state...38
17. Death of a close friend...37
18. Change to different line of work...36
19. Change in frequency of arguments (with spouse)...........................35
20. Large/major mortgage..31
21. Foreclosure of mortgage or loan...30
22. Change in responsibilities at work...29
23. Son or daughter leaving home...29
24. Trouble with in-laws..29
25. Outstanding personal achievement..28
26. Spouse starts or stops work...26
27. Beginning or end of school..26
28. Change in living conditions..25
29. Revision of personal habits..24
30. Trouble with boss...23
31. Change in work hours or conditions..20

32. Change in residence...20
33. Change in schools...20
34. Change in recreation..19
35. Change in church activities...................................19
36. Change in social activities...................................18
37. Minor mortgage or loan..17
38. Change in sleeping habits.....................................16
39. Change in number of family get-togethers....................15
40. Change in eating habits.......................................15
41. Vacaton...13
42. Christas..12
43. Minor violations of the law..................................11

Children also experience stress in many ways. The following list is The Social Readjustment Rating Scale for non-adults (children/ teenagers). Please add up the scores for your child/teenager's life events in the last year.

1. Getting married...101
2. Unwed pregnancy..92
3. Death of a parent..87
4. Acquiring a visible deformity................................81
5. Divorce of parents...77
6. Becoming involved with drugs or alcohol......................76
7. Jail sentence of parent for over one year....................75
8. Marital separation of parents................................69
9. Death of a brother or sister.................................68
10. Change in acceptance by peers................................67
11. Pregnancy of unwed sister....................................64
12. Discovery of being an adopted child..........................63

Definition of Emotion

As stated, stress is defined as a state of worry or mental tension. Mental tension, accompanied by many thoughts of the life event that has caused the stress, then leads to an experience of an emotion. [21] An emotion has been difficult to define over the decades, and still in the 21st century there has been a lot of research and debate among philosophers, historians, psychologists and neuroscientists trying to agree on a definition.[22] The article written by Mulligan & Scherer (2012) in the Journal *Emotion Review*, states that an emotion has several characteristics: an episode in a person's life, has a property of being directed, contains bodily changes such as arousal or expression, can be perceived, involves the person's intellect, and is triggered and guided by the person's cognitive evaluation or interpretation.[23] Emotions occur due to events or situations and last a short time or a long time. For example, sadness is an emotion that often lasts a long time. [24] The Merriam-Webster (2025) definition of emotion is: "a conscious mental reaction, subjectively experienced as a strong feeling, usually directed towards a specific object, and typically accompanied by physiological and behavioural changes."[25] If an emotion is strong or barely controllable, it is called a passion. [26]

As stated, an emotion is subjectively experienced as a strong feeling.[27] Humans feel emotions all over the body. It's commonly known that love is felt over the heart area, and we feel fear in the solar plexus area.[28] Scientists have now discovered that the best way to visualise where someone feels emotions in the body is by thermal imaging or "heat-maps" photographed using thermal cameras.[29] As discussed in the next section, emotions trigger a neurological reaction, and scientists can use an infrared camera to detect specifically where the emotion is felt and where it travels to in the physical body (see Figure 2.1)

.

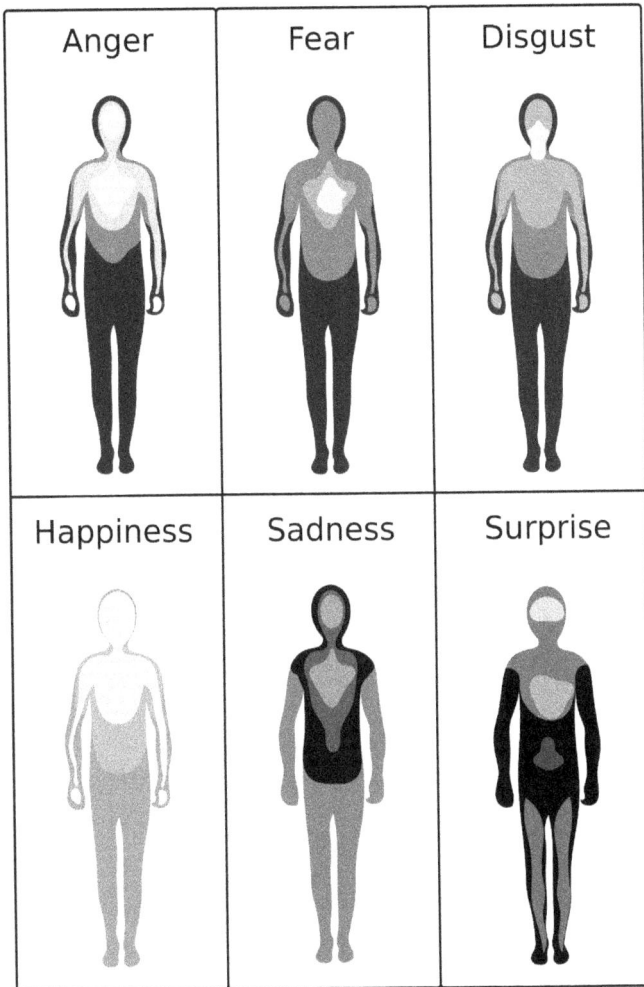

Figure 2.1 Thermal/heat image illustrates where emotions are felt in the human body.

Definition of Anxiety

Anxiety is a brain state that is very often a product of stress and negative emotions.[30] A medical definition of anxiety from the Merriam-

Webster (2025) dictionary is: "an abnormal and overwhelming sense of apprehension and fear often marked by physical signs (such as tension, sweating, and increased pulse rate), by doubt concerning the reality and nature of the threat, and by self-doubt about one's capacity to cope with it."[31] The highlights in this definition are: overwhelming apprehension and fear, and doubt that the self can cope with it, and that there are physical signs that accompany it. [32] This is a very real experience that most people have experienced many times in their lives. The pathway of how thoughts, anxiety, and fear progress to physical stress symptoms will be discussed in the next section of the book. Anxiety becomes an anxiety mental health disorder when it becomes severe and interferes with daily living and can be classified as one of the following: phobias, social anxiety disorder, panic disorder, agoraphobia, generalised anxiety disorder (GAD), separation anxiety disorder, and selective mutism.[33] It is out of the scope of this book to discuss these disorders in detail.

Perception of Stress, Optimism, and Pessimism

The way we perceive a stressful situation can affect our overall well-being and reaction to the situation. Optimism has been strongly associated with better coping skills and quality of life, improved well-being, and decreased mortality.[34] Pessimism is a perceptual trait, like optimism, but is characterised by a negative overall outlook towards life. [35] Optimistic people tend to be more positive and can work through life by setting goals and making plans, and can anticipate positive outcomes. Pessimistic people tend to experience more negative emotions, such as hopelessness or sadness, focus on negative experiences and failures, and expect poor outcomes. [36] Optimism or pessimism can be engrained in our personalities and can be passed on from generation to generation.

On the other hand, people who experience persistent stress and/or long-term exposure to psychological trauma are more likely to develop a pessimistic attitude and be less resilient in the face of adversity. [37]

Physical Stressors

Just as there are psychological stressors that trigger stress, emotions, and anxiety, there are also physical stressors that can cause physical problems within the body. Physical stressors are from physical outside sources, such as the environment, and can also be an internal physical illness. [38] A physical stressor can place physical strain on the body and trigger the stress response. [39] Below is a list of physical stressors:

- Medical procedures (non-surgical)
- Surgery
- Physical trauma, i.e. injury or war
- Medication
- Exertion or sedentary lifestyle
- Pregnancy
- Chemical exposure/pesticides
- Radiation exposure
- Smoking
- Excessive alcohol consumption
- Poor nutrition or malnutrition
- Weather
- Infectious microorganisms (viruses)

How these physical stressors cause problems with our physical health will be explored later. The stress response will now be explained in the following chapter.

Chapter 3

The Stress Response

"Have mercy on me, O LORD, for I am in trouble: my eye wastes away with grief, yes, my soul and my body!"
— Psalm 31:9.

Cumulative or chronic stress is a trigger and an exacerbating factor for many pathological disorders, if left unaddressed, and can consequently result in many life-threatening diseases. These include heart disease, stroke, high blood pressure, diabetes, insomnia, obesity, chronic pain in the body, cardiovascular diseases, depression, and headaches. [40] But how does stress cause these diseases? Let's go back to how Hans Selye discovered the stress response and what it is.

Selye discovered that after rats were exposed to physical stress like cold temperatures, excessive muscular exercise, or surgical injury, or were given intoxicating drugs such as adrenaline or morphine, a "typical syndrome appears."[41] This syndrome would appear regardless of the type of injury or physical stress that the rats were exposed to. [42] The "typical syndrome" was named the "General Adaptation Syndrome" (GAS) and consists of three phases. [43] The first phase is the alarm reaction, the second phase is the resistance phase, and the third phase is the exhaustion phase (Figure 3.1). [44]

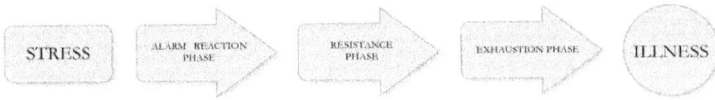

Figure 3.1 General Adaptation Syndrome Phases.

General Adaptation Syndrome Stage One
— The Alarm Reaction and its Neurobiology (The Stress Pathway)

The alarm reaction or alarm stage is when the individual experiences the fight or flight response in the face of a threat, danger or psychological stressor, for example, the sight of a bear, or having an argument with your spouse.[45] The fight or flight response is the stress response in the physical body.[46] In addition, the initial emotion that triggers the fight or flight response is most commonly fear.[47] There is a part of the brain that is the hub of fear and anxiety and, in fact, many negative emotions — it is called the amygdala.[48] The amygdala's name is derived from the Greek word Amygdale, meaning "almond." The reason the old anatomists named the amygdala this is because it is an almond-shaped nucleus deep in the brain (see Figure 3.2). A nucleus in the brain is a cluster of nerve cell bodies. The hippocampus is another cluster of nerve cell bodies that is located close to the amygdala and is also involved in experiencing fear and other emotions, as well as memory formation.[49]

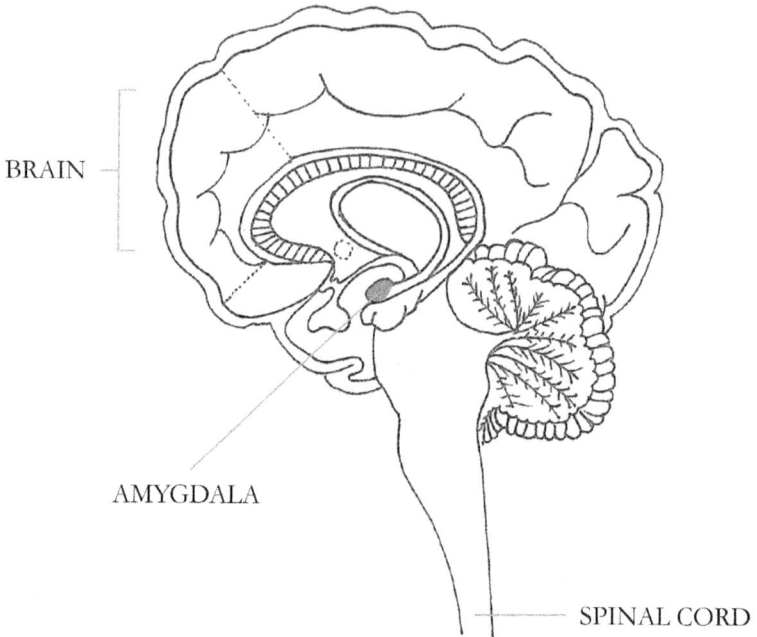

BRAIN

AMYGDALA

SPINAL CORD

Figure 3.2 The Amygdala

When you are confronted with a threat or psychological stressor/ emotional stimulus, like the argument with your spouse example, you see the person and hear their spoken words, and you perceive this sensory experience in the part of the brain called the thalamus, which then communicates to the outer part of the brain called the cortex. Different areas of the cortex that process the visual and auditory (hearing) stimulus communicate with the amygdala, which then triggers your experience of negative emotions such as fear, anxiety, anger and/or sadness.[50] (See Figure 3.3).

CORTEX

THALAMUS
(Perception)

CORTEX
(For Vision)

AMYGDALA
(Emotional Experience)

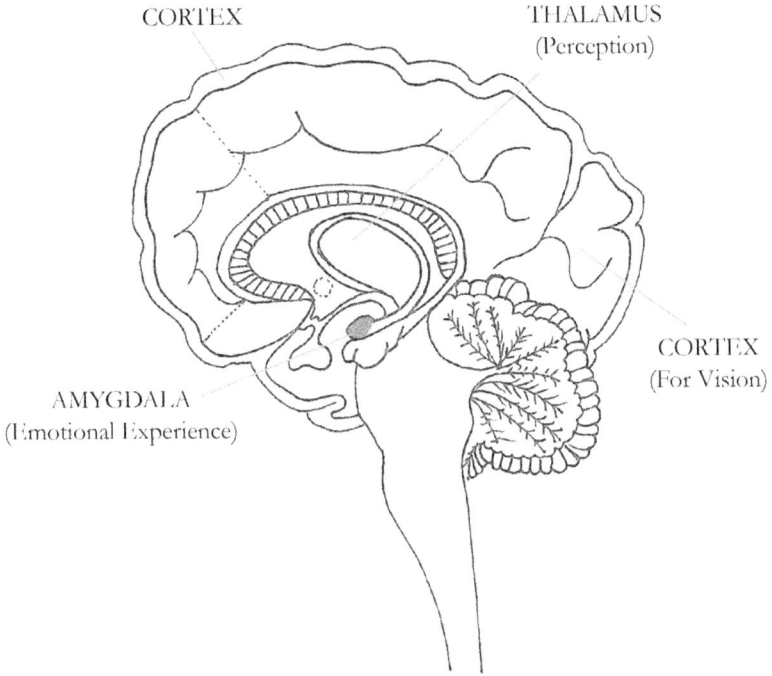

Figure 3.3 The Cortex and Amygdala Connections.

There is an area in the front of the brain (in the frontal cortex) called the ventromedial prefrontal cortex (vmPFC) that can regulate the response of the amygdala.[51] In other words, the vmPFC can suppress the amount of fear or anxiety that we experience.[52]

From the amygdala, there are nerves that travel down to another brain area called the hypothalamus, in particular, an area of the hypothalamus called the paraventricular nucleus (PVN).[53] The hypothalamus is located under the thalamus, as seen in Figure 3.4.

PVN OF HYPOTHALAMUS

THALAMUS

Ventromedial
Prefrontal Cortex

HYPOTHALAMUS

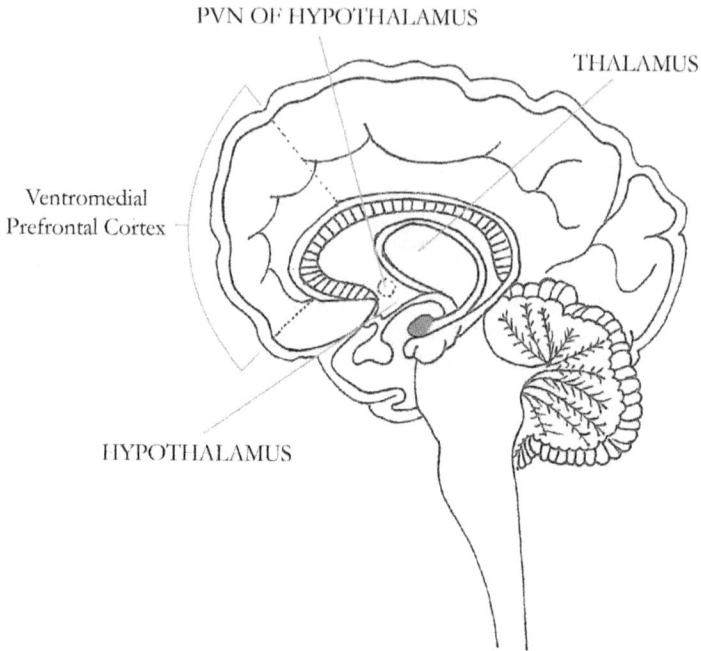

Figure 3.4 The Thalamus, Hypothalamus, and Ventromedial Prefrontal Cortex.

The cells in the PVN of the hypothalamus secrete a hormone called corticotropin-releasing hormone (CRH).[54] CRH travels to the anterior (front part) of the pituitary gland.[55] The pituitary gland is a small pea-sized gland at the base of the brain, as seen in Figure 3.5.

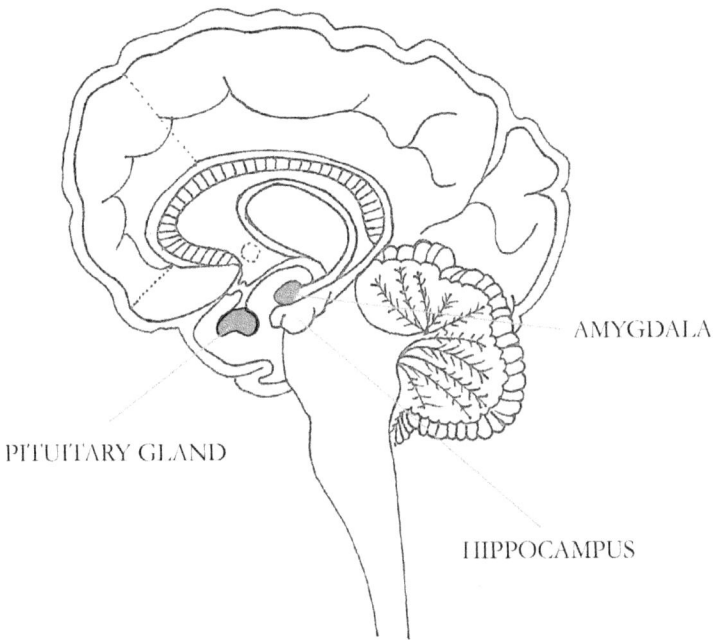

AMYGDALA

PITUITARY GLAND

HIPPOCAMPUS

Figure 3.5 The Pituitary Gland.

In response to CRH, the cells in the anterior pituitary gland release a hormone called adrenocorticotropic hormone (ACTH). [56] This hormone, once released into the bloodstream, travels to the adrenal glands, which are two glands that sit on top of the left and right kidneys.[57] ACTH stimulates the outer layer of the adrenal glands to secrete a steroid hormone called cortisol.[58] You may have heard of cortisol referred to as the stress hormone. Cortisol then travels back through the bloodstream to the brain to stop this stress pathway by way of a structure near the amygdala called the hippocampus.[59] However, if an emotional stimulus is present, the amygdala will continue to trigger this cascade release of hormones where the end point is cortisol release.[60] Cortisol has some very negative effects on the functioning of the human physiology. This entire stress pathway is called the hypothalamic-pituitary-adrenal axis or HPA axis. The pathway is summarised in Figure 3.6.

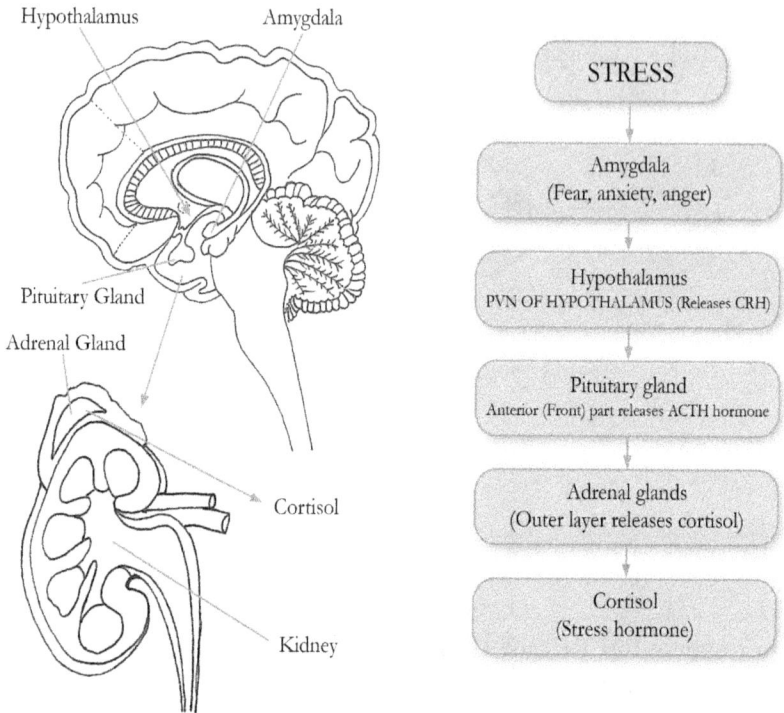

Figure 3.6 The Hypothalamic-Pituitary-Adrenal Axis (HPA Axis) and cortisol.

There is also another pathway of the fight or flight response that does not involve the pituitary gland. This is the sympatho-adrenal-medullary system or SAM system (Figure 3.7). The experience of fear or anxiety from the activation of the amygdala, in the face of physical or psychological stressors, triggers the hypothalamus to then send nerve signals through the brainstem at the base of the brain to the sympathetic nerves.[61] The sympathetic nerves project from the spinal nerves, which exit the spinal cord. Many of the sympathetic nerves end on the adrenal glands. These sympathetic nerves are the only ones that can trigger the release of adrenaline, from the adrenal glands.[62] Adrenaline is a hormone and neurotransmitter that has many effects on the human physiology; some effects are also bad when a person is under prolonged stress.[63] Psychological distress, whether a one-off moment or over frequent episodes, causes activation of the HPA axis by way of the amygdala, as well as activation of the sympatho-adrenal-medullary system, ultimately resulting in concurrent releases of the stress hormone cortisol and adrenaline.[64]

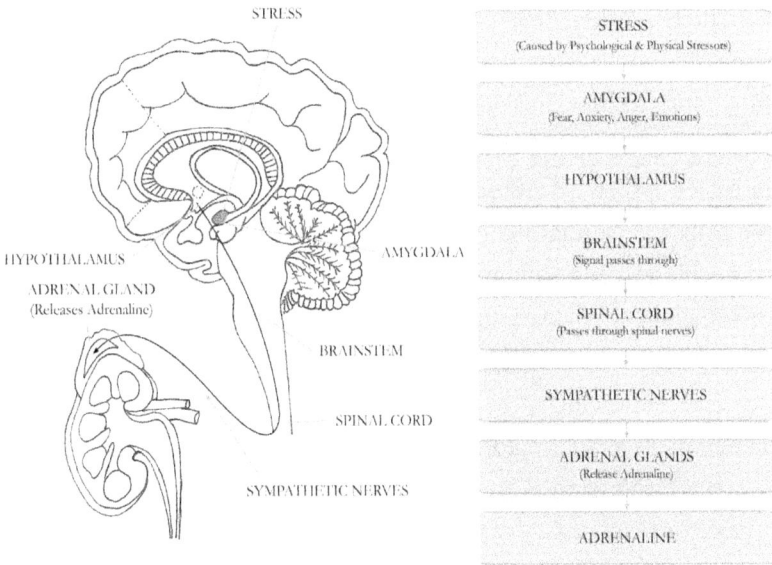

Figure 3.7 The Sympatho-Adrenal-Medullary System and Adrenaline.

Hans Selye found that during this general adaptation stage one, certain organs of the body were affected. He found that the organs of the thymus, spleen, and other immune glands, which make our immune cells, shrank.[65] He found that the liver shrank, there was a disappearance of fat tissue and loss of muscular tone, and that erosions began to form in the digestive tract, particularly the stomach, small intestine, and the appendix.[66] Selye found that this occurred regardless of the type of stressor, physical or psychological.[67]

Nowadays, after many years of research since Selye's experimentation, it is known how these physiological effects come about in the organs. Some of these effects can be explained by exploring what cortisol and adrenaline do.

Effects of Adrenaline on the Body

Adrenaline has a wide range of effects on the body under stressful conditions. Adrenaline can increase fat tissue breakdown, and it opens the airways to increase oxygen in the body, causes the heart to contract harder and quicker, and increases the release of glucose in the liver so that a person has enough "energy" to run from the threat or stressor. [68] Adrenaline also decreases insulin released from the pancreas, so that the blood sugar remains high. [69] The number of white blood cells (immune cells) increases initially after exposure to adrenaline; however, their responsiveness to a pathogen such as a virus or bacteria is reduced. [70]

The following is a list of health conditions where excess adrenaline is a contributor:[71]

- Depression
- Anxiety
- Irritable Bowel Syndrome
- Hypertension
- Diabetes
- Weight problems
- Ageing
- Insomnia
- Restless Leg Syndrome
- Headaches
- Addictions
- Urinary urgency and Bed-Wetting

- Fibromyalgia
- Urinary Tract Infections
- Road Rage
- Bipolar Disorder
- Hyperemesis Gravidarum (nausea during pregnancy)
- Cyclical Vomiting Syndrome
- Autism
- ADHD
- Post-Traumatic Stress Disorder
- Premenstrual Dysphoric Disorder

Effects of Cortisol on the Body

Cortisol is a natural steroid hormone that controls the sleep-wake cycle called the circadian rhythm and has multiple other roles in the body. Normal cortisol levels are increased by chronic stress, and this can consequently increase blood pressure, decrease oestrogen and testosterone levels, and cause shrinking of the immune system tissues, essentially suppressing the immune cells and causing inflammation.[72] Moreover, inflammation in the body is caused by chronically elevated cortisol levels due to persistent and ongoing stress.[73] An example of the relationship between stress and inflammation caused by cortisol is that people who have suffered trauma and have consequently developed post-traumatic stress disorder (PTSD) are more likely to have elevated inflammatory molecules and, consequently, chronic conditions that are commonly associated with PTSD.[74] There is growing evidence that chronic inflammation in the human body, caused by stress and elevated cortisol, has a contributing effect on the development of non-communicable/chronic diseases such as cardiovascular disease (heart disease that can lead to heart attack), cancer, stroke, neurodegenerative disorders such as Alzheimer's disease and Parkinson's disease, and psychological disorders such as depression.[75]

General Adaptation Syndrome Stage Two
— The Resistance Phase

The resistance or adaptation phase starts with the actions of cortisol and adrenaline as they continue to be secreted due to the persistent stressor.[76] The key feature of the resistance phase is that the body resists the continuous effects of the stressor and the effects of cortisol and adrenaline, and when the stressor has passed, the person's body will find a new equilibrium by adjusting to the new environment. [77] All people go through the alarm phase and the resistance phase many times in their lives, as there will always be stressors that will challenge the body. [78] Without these first two phases, humans would not continue to evolve. [79]

General Adaptation Syndrome Stage Three
— The Exhaustion Phase

If a stressor is persistent and the stress the individual perceives is prolonged and intense, the individual's body will move into the exhaustion phase. [80] In this exhaustion phase, the body's ability to respond to the continuous stressor, and new stressors, is greatly impaired. The "load" of stress on the body that is formally named "allostatic load" becomes too much. [81] The stress hormones cortisol and adrenaline remain chronically elevated and the body experiences illness. The ability of the body to shut off the stress response when the stressor is eliminated is decreased.[82] An individual may experience conditions such as persistent high blood pressure (hypertension), high blood sugar, and a diagnosis of diabetes or even cancer. This is because the immune system, which is not functioning strongly, can't destroy cancer cells that are formed (we all make cancer cells, but the immune system destroys them when we are healthy). [83]

Selye theorised that stress could cause disease, and this is now widely accepted as being a reality.[84] It is now known that a wide range of diseases, acute, chronic and life-threatening, such as cardiovascular disease, stroke, diabetes, and cancer, are caused by the inflammation that occurs because of chronic stress.[85]

Other Body Axes Affected Under Stress

The HPA axis is not the only axis that is affected by stress. The hypothalamic-pituitary-gonadal axis (HPG axis) and the hypothalamic-pituitary-thyroid axis (HPT axis) are also affected. The HPG axis is influenced by the HPA axis and, as a result, causes suppression of the release of oestrogen and testosterone from the ovaries and testes, respectively.[86] Essentially, stress, when chronic, can cause decreased function of the gonads, leading to problems such as infertility in both men and women and changes in menstruation in women.[87] Specifically, chronic stress decreases spermatogenesis, which is the production of sperm in men, and can disrupt or stop ovulation in women and, therefore, can delay menstruation, causing irregular periods.[88] Chronic stress causes the hypothalamic-pituitary-thyroid axis to decrease production of thyroid hormones, contributing to conditions such as autoimmune hypothyroidism, where the thyroid gland that sits in the front of your neck area does not function optimally (Figure 3.8).[89] Please see Figure 3.9 for a chapter summary.

Figure 3.8 The Hypothalamic-Pituitary-Gonadal Axis (HPG Axis) and the

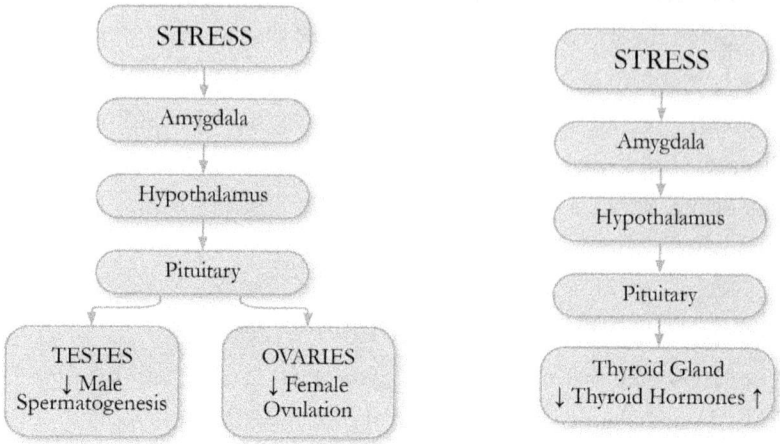

Hypothalamic-Pituitary-Thyroid Axis (HPT Axis)

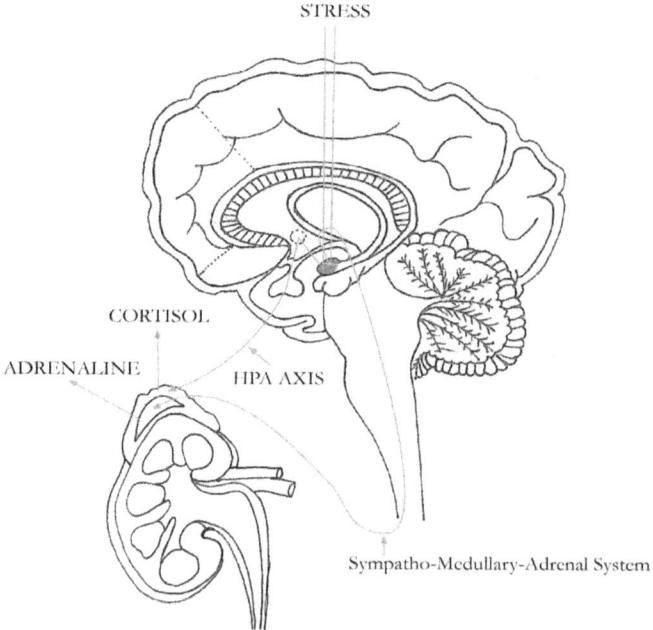

Figure 3.9 Chapter Summary

Chapter 4

The Effect of Physical Stressors
on the Body

As stated in Chapter 2, a physical stressor can place physical strain on the body and trigger the stress response.[90] Below is an outline of how these stressors can affect our health.

Medical Procedures (Non-Surgical), Surgery, Physical Trauma

Stress is essential to survival and aids the human organism in surviving physical trauma. However, physical stress, such as surgery or a physical injury, can be harmful, adding to the severity of an existing medical problem or creating new stress-related medical conditions.[91] Some overt acute stressors, such as physical traumas (injury or surgery), can cause post-traumatic stress disorder, a severe inflammatory response, deep vein thrombosis (blood clots in the veins of the legs), pulmonary embolism (blood clots in the lungs), myocardial infarction (heart attack), life-threatening arrhythmias (irregular heart beat), and sudden cardiac death. [92] Also, stress experienced before a surgery related to fear of anaesthetic, psychological fear of the surgery failing to help, and even fear of the unknown, can lead to complications in surgical procedures and can prolong recovery.[93]

Furthermore, studies in the field of children who must undergo surgery or invasive medical procedures (such as in an intensive care unit) have shown that these children may experience fear, post-traumatic stress disorder, re-experiencing the event, hyper-arousal, and avoidance behaviours.[94] This can lead to developmental delays, impairment in social and scholastic functioning, difficulties sleeping, and mood disturbances.[95]

Medication

It is well known among medical and nursing professionals that all medications can have unwanted side effects and adverse reactions in many individuals, and may cause injury to the liver and kidneys, where all drugs are metabolised.[96] For example, second-generation antipsychotic medications are known to cause metabolic and inflammatory side effects such as weight gain, metabolic syndrome, diabetes mellitus, cardiovascular disease, acute kidney injury, chronic kidney disease, and liver damage.[97] Another example is that chronic opioid use is known to cause liver damage.[98] It is not necessary to give examples of all drug groups and their side effects, but it is good to be aware that all medications can have an effect on the liver and kidneys, which are the central organs of their metabolism.[99]

Exertion and a Sedentary Lifestyle

When an individual exercises, a multitude of changes occur to the immune system and the neuroendocrine/hormonal system.[100] In general, moderate exercise is associated with an improved state of health. However, overexertion (exercise that is too intense) may lead to illness as it triggers the stress response, leading to increased cortisol production and suppression of the immune system. Heart arrhythmias can occur due to exertion.[101] On the other hand, a sedentary lifestyle where an individual does not exercise at all may also lead to illness, as there are fewer immune cells overall in this group of people.[102]

Pregnancy

Pregnancy can affect the health of both the mother's physical body and her mental health. Women can potentially suffer multimorbidity during pregnancy, such as physical, psychological, and social ill health.[103] Common perinatal mental health disorders are anxiety, depression, and somatic disorders, such as experiencing stress and anxiety due to the physical changes to the body during pregnancy.[104]

For every maternal death due to pregnancy complications, 20 to 30 women are estimated to have illnesses related to pregnancy or childbirth.[105] Pregnancy can cause gestational diabetes due to a complex interplay of hormones that cause insulin resistance.[106] Maternal weight gain is problematic for a woman. Not only is a heavier body weight stigmatised globally, particularly in advanced economies, but it is also associated with depression and experiences of overeating, decreased exercise motivation, and more unhealthy food choices.[107] Consequently, experiences of weight gain stigma are associated with increased weight gain and obesity over time.[108] The experience of weight gain stigma causes stress and, therefore, elevated cortisol levels, which have an array of effects on the body as previously discussed. [109] Weight gain during pregnancy is often permanent and is associated with other chronic diseases, such as high blood pressure and post-natal depression. [110]

Radiation Exposure

Ionising radiation is defined as energy released by atoms in the form of electromagnetic waves.[111] The electromagnetic spectrum is shown below in Figure 4.1. All energy that is emitted from a source is radiation on the electromagnetic spectrum, including visible light, the sun (Ultraviolet light), microwaves, radio waves or X-rays.[112] Higher-frequency electromagnetic waves are X-rays and gamma rays. [113] This type of radiation can "ionise" an atom; in other words, it can remove an electron from an atom in your cells. [114] Gamma rays, which are the highest-frequency radiation, are able to damage living cells and transfer energy from one cell to another.[115] Lower-frequency electromagnetic waves do not have as much energy and do not ionise atoms, and therefore are less harmful to humans. [116]

Figure 4.1 Diagram of the Different Types of Radiation.

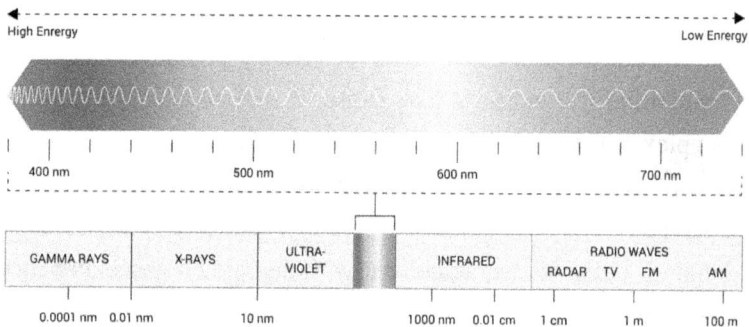

Another form of radiation that is ionising is emitted from particles such as alpha, beta, and neutron particles and is called particulate radiation. [117] These particles carry an electrical charge and can directly affect atoms in cells. Soil, water, food, and the Earth all emit ionising radiation in the form of either gamma rays, alpha, beta, or neutron particles. [118] A person on earth is exposed to an average of 2.4 mSv (millisieverts) per year of ionising radiation; however, this may vary in different countries. [119] A high dose of ionising radiation can cause acute disease presentations such as skin burns, hair loss, or a condition called acute radiation syndrome. This syndrome may occur when someone is treated with radiation for the medical treatment of cancer. [120] Low doses of ionising radiation over time may lead to chronic conditions such as cancer. This is because the radiation can damage cells through what is known as "oxidative stress," leading to the replication of damaged cells that eventuate into a tumour/cell mass. [121] The cancer may appear decades after repeated radiation exposure.[122] Cancer risk may occur when an individual is exposed to 100 mSv.[123]

Chemicals and Pesticides

Artificial chemicals and pesticides have been used extensively worldwide and are hazardous to the environment and human health.[124] Chemicals that are absorbed in various ways, such as orally, through inhalation, and through absorption through the skin, are contributors to the development of chronic disease. This can be life-threatening, should the disease become acute.[125] The way in which chemicals influence the development of chronic disease remains unclear to researchers at this time.[126] However, once the chemical is absorbed into the tissues of the body, it travels through the bloodstream and can have a detrimental effect on various organs.[127] For example, chemicals have been proven to contribute to the development of diabetes, cancers, chronic nervous system diseases, cardiovascular disease, obesity, increased cholesterol levels, high blood pressure, thyroid disease, and male and female reproductive disorders.[128] Many chemicals particularly disrupt the endocrine system, causing hormone-sensitive cancers and diseases such as polycystic ovarian syndrome and endometriosis.[129] For example, females with endometriosis have higher levels of Bisphenol A (BPA) in their urine.[130] BPA is a synthetic chemical used to synthesise epoxy resins, polymer materials, and polycarbonate plastics, which can be found in food containers, water and baby bottles, toys, paints, sports equipment, medical devices, and the lining of canned foods.[131] BPA causes carcinogenesis (development of cancer), suppresses the immune system, disrupts the endocrine system and causes infertility.[132] Other chemicals that are particularly hazardous are: plasticisers, pesticides, flame retardants, environmental pollutants in food, and surfactants.[133]

Particulate Matter (PM), a mixture of chemicals and biological elements, is found in air pollution and is also a cause of chronic non-communicable diseases worldwide.[134] PM is a risk factor for contracting chronic conditions such as lung cancer, asthma, chronic obstructive pulmonary disease (COPD), cardiovascular disease, high blood pressure, heart attack (myocardial infarction), stroke, loss of cognitive function, anxiety, Parkinson's and Alzheimer's diseases. [135] Its main hallmark is that PM causes chronic inflammation that contributes to the development of these diseases. [136]

Heavy metal (HM) poisoning is a huge risk to human health worldwide.[137] The main heavy metals that can reach toxic levels in the human body are chromium, arsenic, nickel, cadmium, lead, mercury, zinc, and copper. [138] These heavy metals are present in food (grains, fruit, vegetables, seafood, and poultry), water, soil (fertilisers and pesticides), and the air. HMs have been associated with harm to the kidneys, brain, intestines, lungs, liver, and bones, causing cancer and imbalances to the immune system. [139] Even trace amounts of HMs are toxic to human health. [140]

Poor Nutrition or Malnutrition

Poor nutrition is associated with the risk of chronic disease over the lifespan.[141] Obesity is a risk factor for chronic diseases in children and adults.[142] Often, poor food choices lead to malnutrition and vitamin/protein deficiencies, as the food that is consumed has little nutritional value and, when consumed, becomes a physical stressor on the body rather than beneficial. Examples of these are foods such as packaged candy, biscuits, chips, fast-food, refined grains such as white bread/rice/pasta; basically, any food source that contains ultra-processed food that is high in salt, trans fats, added sugar, stabilisers, and preservatives.[143] There is evidence in the literature that a diet high in red meat, refined carbohydrates, and saturated fat is pro-inflammatory, and a diet high in fruit, vegetables, legumes, wholegrains, nuts, spices, herbs and plant-based protein is anti-inflammatory.[144] Adequate nutrition is imperative to maintaining good immunity, not only for children and adults, but also for the frail elderly, who are already in a state of age-related inflammation.[145]

Smoking

Smoking is responsible for over 175 million deaths worldwide over the past three decades.[146] Tobacco cigarettes contain nicotine; however, tobacco cigarettes, e-cigarettes, and waterpipes such as shisha all contain an array of chemicals such as formaldehyde, lead, carbon monoxide, and particulate matter, which are all toxic to humans.[147] Nicotine increases blood pressure and heart rate. It contains chemical compounds that are confirmed in the research to cause inflammation, cancer (predominantly head and neck cancer and lung cancer), and other diseases such as cardiovascular disease and chronic lung diseases, as well as impairment in cognitive ability.[148]

Excessive Alcohol Consumption

Harmful or excessive use of alcohol is a physical stressor and contributes to 2.6 million deaths per year globally.[149] Excessive alcohol is also responsible for the disabilities and poor health of millions of people, as it is a risk factor for many acute and chronic diseases.[150] Alcohol is classed as a Group 1 carcinogen, which means that it is confirmed to be a cause of cancer in humans, as stated by the International Agency for Research on Cancer.[151] According to the World Health Organisation (2023), alcohol is known to cause at least seven different types of cancer, including bowel cancer and breast cancer.[152] Alcohol is a risk factor for foetal alcohol syndrome, epilepsy, liver cirrhosis and pancreatitis, diabetes, cardiovascular disease, high blood pressure (hypertension), ischaemic heart disease (where the heart's arteries are blocked with plaque that can lead to a heart attack), stroke, and cardiac arrhythmias.[153]

Weather

Weather changes have the potential to affect human health and are therefore a physical stressor.[154] There is growing global evidence that climate change is having damaging effects on human living conditions, as well as physical and mental health. [155] Climate change is significantly increasing the incidence of infectious diseases, particularly vector-borne diseases such as those transmitted by mosquitoes in places such as Asia, sub-Saharan Africa, and South America.[156] The incidence of infectious diseases caused by viruses, bacteria, fungi, and parasites can be influenced by fluctuating weather patterns.[157]

In Traditional Chinese Medicine, six Pernicious Influences exist, which are known as climatic phenomena.[158] The Pernicious Influences are Wind, Cold, Fire or Heat, Dampness, Dryness, and Summer Heat, and can change the internal state of the body, predisposing a person to an acute disease state. [159]

Furthermore, people with chronic pain, such as those who suffer from chronic conditions such as rheumatoid arthritis, phantom limb syndrome, scar pain, trigeminal neuralgia, lower back pain, and headaches/migraines, frequently report that their pain is worse when there are changes in the weather.[160] Weather conditions that can trigger the worsening of pain symptoms are: humidity, thunderstorms, cold temperatures, barometric pressure, precipitation, and sunshine. [161]

Viruses

Viruses are being proven to predispose people to certain cancers and are therefore a physical stressor on the human body. One of the best examples of this is the human papillomavirus, or HPV, which is sexually transmitted even with only skin-to-skin contact.[162] Approximately 99.7% of cervical cancer cases are caused by an infection with HPV.[163] The virus infects the cells in the cervix and disrupts normal cell division, leading to abnormal cancer cells that multiply into lesions.[164]

Liver cancer, also known as hepatocellular carcinoma (HCC), is one of the leading causes of death from cancer worldwide.[165] The major causes of liver cancer are hepatitis B and C viral infections, which are predominant in China and other Asian countries such as Japan, Korea and Taiwan, Africa, and also in high-income countries such as the United States.[166] Hepatitis B virus can cause alterations in the liver cells' genetic programming and immune cell reactions to the liver cells. This, coupled with other stressors or risk factors such as diabetes, obesity, or excessive alcohol consumption, can result in liver damage, called liver cirrhosis, and consequently contribute to liver cancer.[167]

Chapter 5

The Mind-Body and Brain-Body Connection

It is now widely known among clinicians and researchers that mental and physical health are closely connected.[168] Researchers have found that mental and physical illnesses often occur at the same time and that stress and adverse experiences pose adverse physical health outcomes, through a variety of mechanisms that we have explored so far in this book.[169] There is a strong connection between the mind-brain-body and the body-brain-mind, in particular, the relationship between the brain and the immune system and the gut immune system, called the gut microbiome.[170]

The Brain and the Immune System are Connected

It was explained in Chapter 3 that stressors perceived by the brain can trigger the cascade of events that ends in the release of cortisol and adrenaline from the adrenal glands. Too much cortisol and adrenaline can trigger intricate connections and chemical reactions in the immune cells and suppress their function. The immune system is also connected to the brain.[171] As the growth of infectious bacteria or viruses increases, the immune response is to signal the brain to produce a fever.[172] A fever is a state of hyperthermia, where the rising temperature is designed to kill microorganisms.[173]

What is the Gut Microbiome?

The gut microbiome is a high-density abundance of microbes or "flora," which exist in the gastrointestinal tract of humans and animals and is both natural and important for our overall well-being.[174] The microbiome in the gut is composed of bacteria from the Firmicutes, Bacteroidetes, Actinobacteria, Fusobacteria, Proteobacteria, and Verrucomicrobia phyla.[175] These microbes are high in numbers and outnumber human cells.[176] Certain dietary patterns can affect the gut microbiome across a lifespan. It is beneficial to eat fibre in the form of fruit, vegetables, and wholegrains, which promote diverse and beneficial gut microbiota.[177] It is harmful to consume foods that are physical stressors, such as refined sugars/carbohydrates, fats, and any processed foods. Overconsumption of these foods causes a condition called dysbiosis, which is characterised by a reduction in microbial diversity and an increase in harmful bacteria in the intestines.[178] This increase in harmful bacteria can contribute to obesity, inflammation, and chronic metabolic disorders.[179]

The Relationship Between the Brain, Stress, Immune System, and the Gut Microbiome

The gut microbiome influences the brain through the gut-brain axis.[180] The gut-brain axis is the connection between the nerves in the gut and the nerves that then travel back to the brain.[181] Therefore, the state of our natural gut microbiome influences our brain and can affect mental health.[182] There is increasing evidence in the literature that suggests that the composition of our gut microbiome has a strong influence on the development of depression and anxiety.[183] Additionally, depression and anxiety disorders are heavily influenced by stress and the HPA axis, which can also be beneficially modified by a healthy gut microbiome.[184] Therefore, stress and inflammation negatively influencing the gut microbiome play a role in the development of anxiety and depression.[185] The gut microbiota, in fact, plays a role in many diseases, including cancer.[186] A dysbiosis predisposes an individual to increased chronic inflammation and a decreased immune response to cancer cells, allowing the cells to increase in number without a healthy immune system to destroy them. [187]

Have You Ever Heard of... "Psychosomatic?"

A psychosomatic reaction is a physical reaction or response to a psychological stressor, or in other words, a mental or emotional disturbance.[188] A good example of this can be seen in victims of bullying. Bullying is traumatic and can cause psychological stress. Victims of childhood bullying have been found to develop common physical illnesses such as colds, but also psychosomatic problems such as headaches, stomach aches, and sleeping problems, and commonly take up smoking in their teenage or adult years.[189] Also, children and adults who are bullied are more likely to develop internalisation of psychological stress and develop anxiety and depression disorders. [190] Adult victims of bullying also find that they experience more frequent headaches, poor general health, including more bodily pain, and slower recovery from illnesses. [191]

Functional gastrointestinal (GI) disorders are a group of disorders, such as irritable bowel syndrome (IBS) and functional dyspepsia (FD), that are characterised by abdominal symptoms; however, there is no actual structural cause for them.[192] These conditions have been classed as completely psychosomatic until recently, with research increasingly showing that sufferers also have gut dysbiosis and altered immune reactions or hypersensitivity to certain foods.[193] However, many of the symptoms, such as abdominal pain, originate from psychological stressors coupled with anxiety, depression, and altered brain processing. [194]

Functional neurological disorder (FND) is a condition characterised by an abnormality in brain networks and connections rather than in brain structures.[195] The symptoms involve a sudden and unexpected deterioration in physical functioning or movement, to the point where the sufferer cannot move or has symptoms of dystonia, an abnormality in muscle tone. [196] Much research has shown that there are certain brain areas in patients with FND that are activated, but not diseased. [197] The amygdala — remember that almond-shaped area of the brain that is involved in stress, anxiety, and fear? In FND sufferers, the amygdala is abnormally activated, and this precedes the person's deterioration in movement, as it causes the area of the brain involved in physical movement to shut off (primary motor cortex). [198] Researchers have found that the increased activation of the amygdala in response to psychological stressors should be the focus of study for future treatment of FND. [199]

Chapter 6

Stress, Allostatic Load, and Recommendations

Allostasis is the term that describes a person's ability to experience stability amidst repeated change and challenges, both psychological and physical. Allostasis is really Stage two of the General Adaptation Syndrome — the resistance phase. The body achieves a state of balance where the stressors impacting the affected person fail to cause exhaustion and illness. Instead, they contribute to the growth of the individual and they achieve a new "normal." This is healthy functioning.[200]

McEwan and Stellar introduced the concept of allostatic load in 1993.[201] Allostatic load is the accumulation of stressful ordinary life events, significant life events, such as those in the SRRS in Chapter 2, and physical stressors that are perceived as stressful and beyond the person's ability to cope.[202] The person's body enters the exhaustion phase, where the excessive activation of the HPA axis results in chronically elevated cortisol, and adrenaline predominates.

It seems that the start of cancer, a stroke, heart disease, autoimmune disease, and other illnesses begins after a significant or stressful life event.[203] Where can you go from here?

Recommendations for Healing

It is recommended to treat illness holistically by using a combination of Eastern and Western medicine, or in other words, modern medicine and complementary therapies.[204] The following are some ways to reduce stress levels. It is important to consult your doctor if you are experiencing symptoms that are impacting your well-being and mental or physical health.

- Activate the parasympathetic nervous system with relaxation/meditation/mindfulness.
- Practise forgiveness of yourself and others.
- Release emotional stress in a healthy way, such as journalling.
- Get out of your head and into your body by taking a walk, swimming, practising yoga, dancing, getting a massage, or getting among nature.
- Seek a qualified counsellor or psychologist if needed.
- Nourish your body, which is your temple, with whole foods and plenty of fibre such as fruit and vegetables (ideally organic), which are rich in antioxidants.
- Try consulting a complementary therapy specialist such as a naturopath, chiropractor, physiotherapist, herbal therapist, flower essence therapist, or healer.
- Have alcohol in moderation, and limit or quit smoking and recreational drugs.
- Keep connected to your family and friends and nurture those relationships.
- Get good quality sleep.

The following quote summarises a healthy outlook that we must strive for to flourish in our lives in the 21st century, as stressful as life is for many of us:

To flourish requires more than being physically healthy, it requires that we make significant strides toward fulfilling our dreams and aspirations as productive people, that we be viewed as cherished friends, counted as valued community members and, at the end of our lives, find some comfort and satisfaction in the important personal work of establishing who we are and finding meaning in why we were here. To accomplish these ends is to lead a balanced, resilient life, and as research in psychoneuroimmunology shows, one that has decreased illness and greater longevity.

— Quote taken from Christiansen (2007)[205]

Endnotes

1   Oxford English Dictionary. (n.d.). Disease, N. In *Oed.com.* Retrieved December 2024, from *disease, n. meanings, etymology and more | Oxford English Dictionary*

2   Oxford English Dictionary. (n.d.). Disease, N. In *Oed.com.* Retrieved December 2024, from *disease, n. meanings, etymology and more | Oxford English Dictionary*

3   Singh, H. (2024). *Public health: A global perspective.* Productivity Press.

4   McCance, K. L., & Heuther, S. E. (2019). *Pathophysiology: The biologic basis for disease in adults and children.* (8th e.d.). Mosby.

5   McCance, K. L., & Heuther, S. E. (2019). *Pathophysiology: The biologic basis for disease in adults and children.* (8th e.d.). Mosby.

6   Manning, E., & Gagnon, M. (2017). The complex patient: A concept clarification. *Nursing and Health Sciences, 19,* 13-21. https://doi.org/10.1111/nhs.12320

7   Manning, E., & Gagnon, M. (2017). The complex patient: A concept clarification. *Nursing and Health Sciences, 19,* 13-21. https://doi.org/10.1111/nhs.12320

8   Lynch, J., & Davey Smith, G. (2005). A life course approach to chronic disease epidemiology. *Annual Review of Public Health, 26,* 1-35. https://doi.org/10.1146/annurev.publhealth.26.021304.144505

9   Manning, E., & Gagnon, M. (2017). The complex patient: A concept clarification. *Nursing and Health Sciences, 19,* 13-21. https://doi.org/10.1111/nhs.12320

10   Varona, P., Bonet, M., Garcia, R., Chang, M., Suarez, R., & National Provincial Coordinating Group. Implementation of chronic disease risk factor surveillance in 12 Cuban municipalities. *MEDICC Review, 14*(1), 43-47.

11   Mrazek, P.J., & Haggerty, R.J. (1994). *Reducing risks for*

mental disorders: Frontiers for preventive intervention research. National Academies Press.

12 Pietrzak, R. H., Goldstein, R. B., Southwick, S. M., & Grant, B. F. (2012). Physical health conditions associated with posttraumatic stress disorder in U.S. older adults: Results from wave 2 of the National Epidemiologic Survey on Alcohol and Related Conditions. *Journal of the American Geriatrics Society, 60*(2), 296-303. https://doi.org/10.1111/j.1532-5415.2011.03788.x

13 Christiansen, C. (2007). Adolf Meyer revisited: Connections between lifestyles, resilience and illness. *Journal of Occupational Science, 14*(2), 63–76. https://doi.org/10.1080/14427591.2007.9686586

14 World Health Organisation. (2023). *Stress.* Stress

15 Jackson, M. (2014). Evaluating the role of Hans Selye in the modern history of stress. In D. Cantor & E. Ramsden, *Stress, Shock, and Adaptation in the Twentieth Century.* (pp. 21-48). University of Rochester Press.

16 Jackson, M. (2014). Evaluating the Role of Hans Selye in the modern history of stress. In D. Cantor & E. Ramsden, *Stress, Shock, and Adaptation in the Twentieth Century.* (pp. 21-48). University of Rochester Press; Rochette, L., Dogon, G., & Vergely, C. (2023). Stress: Eight decades after its definition by Hans Selye: "Stress is the Spice of Life." *Brain Sciences, 13*(310), 1-3. https://doi.org/10.3390/brainsci13020310; Zimbardo, G., Johnson, R. L., & McCann V. (2012) *General adaptation syndrome: Hans Selye.* Essay; Ramanathan, R., & Desrouleaux, R. (2022). Introduction: The science of stress. *Yale Journal of Biology & Medicine, 95*(1), 1-2. https://pmc.ncbi.nlm.nih.gov/articles/PMC8961711/

17 Agorastos, A., & Chrousos, G. P. (2022). The neuroendocrinology of stress: the stress related continuum of chronic disease development. *Molecular Psychiatry, 27,* 502-513. https://doi.org/10.1038/s41380-021-01224-9

18   Davis, A. E., Nathanson, J., Attwood. K., Sinha, A. A., Seiffert-Sinha, K. (2024). A retrospective analysis of patient-reported physical and psychological stressors as trigger factors in autoimmune bullous disease. *Archives of Dermatological Research, 316*(515), 1-4. https://doi.org/10.1007/s00403-024-03240-5

19   Hechtman, L. (2012). *Clinical naturopathic medicine.* Elsevier Australia.

20   Hechtman, L. (2012). *Clinical naturopathic medicine.* Elsevier Australia.

21   World Health Organisation. (2023). *Stress. Stress*

22   Hartmann, K. (2024). Understanding the language: Key features of emotions. *Acta Psychologica, 251*(104628), 1-11. https://doi.org/10.1016/j.actpsy.2024.104628

23   Mulligan, K., & Scherer, K. R. (2012). Toward a working definition of emotion. *Emotion Review, 4*(4), 345-357. https://doi.org/10.1177/1754073912445818

24   Mulligan, K., & Scherer, K. R. (2012). Toward a working definition of emotion. *Emotion Review, 4*(4), 345-357. https://doi.org/10.1177/1754073912445818

25   Merriam-Webster, Incorporated. (n.d.). Emotion. In *Merriam-Webster Dictionary.* Retrieved 2025, from *EMOTION Definition & Meaning - Merriam-Webster*

26   Merriam-Webster, Incorporated. (n.d.). Emotion. In *Merriam-Webster Dictionary.* Retrieved 2025, from *EMOTION Definition & Meaning - Merriam-Webster*

27   Merriam-Webster, Incorporated. (n.d.). Emotion. In *Merriam-Webster Dictionary.* Retrieved 2025, from *EMOTION Definition & Meaning - Merriam-Webster*

28   Myss, C. (1996). *Anatomy of the spirit: The seven stages of power & healing.* Transworld Publishers.

29   Ilikci, B., Chen, L., Cho, H., & Liu, Q. (2019). Heat-map based emotion and face recognition from thermal images. *IEEE,* 449-

453. https://doi.org/10.1109/ComComAp46287.2019.9018786

30 Tovote, P., Fadok, J. P., & Lüthi, A. (2015). Neural circuits for fear and anxiety. *Nature Reviews Neuroscience, 16,* 317-331. https://doi.org/10.1038/nrn3945

31 Merriam-Webster, Incorporated. (n.d.). Anxiety. In *Merriam-Webster Dictionary.* Retrieved 2025, from *ANXIETY Definition & Meaning - Merriam-Webster*

32 Merriam-Webster, Incorporated. (n.d.). Anxiety. In *Merriam-Webster Dictionary.* Retrieved 2025, from *ANXIETY Definition & Meaning - Merriam-Webster*

33 Domschke, K., Seuling, P. D., Schiele, M. A., Bandelow, B., Batelaan, N. M., Bokma, W. A., Branchi, I., Broich, K., Burkauskas, J., Davies, S. J. C., Dell'Osso, B., Fagan, H., Fineberg, N.A., Furukawa, T. A., Hofmann, S. G., Hood, S., Huneke, N. T. M., Latas, M., Lidbetter, N., ... Baldwin, D. S. (2024). The definition of treatment resistance in anxiety disorders: a Delphi method-based consensus guideline. *World Psychiatry, 23*(1), 113-123. https://doi.org/10.1002/wps.21177

34 Paat, Y., Hope, T. L., Ferreira-Pinto, J. B., & Alvarez, H. O. (2024). A bio-psycho-social approach to understanding optimism and pessimism in response to stress. European Journal of Investigation in Health, Psychology and Education, 14(10), 2671-2685. https://doi.org/10.3390/ejihpe14100176

35 Paat, Y., Hope, T. L., Ferreira-Pinto, J. B., & Alvarez, H. O. (2024). A bio-psycho-social approach to understanding optimism and pessimism in response to stress. European Journal of Investigation in Health, Psychology and Education, 14(10), 2671-2685. https://doi.org/10.3390/ejihpe14100176

36 Paat, Y., Hope, T. L., Ferreira-Pinto, J. B., & Alvarez, H. O. (2024). A bio-psycho-social approach to understanding optimism and pessimism in response to stress. European Journal of Investigation in Health, Psychology and Education, 14(10), 2671-2685. https://doi.

org/10.3390/ejihpe14100176

37 Paat, Y., Hope, T. L., Ferreira-Pinto, J. B., & Alvarez, H. O. (2024). A bio-psycho-social approach to understanding optimism and pessimism in response to stress. European Journal of Investigation in Health, Psychology and Education, 14(10), 2671-2685. https://doi.org/10.3390/ejihpe14100176

38 Daviu, N., Bruchas, M. R., Moghaddam, B., Sandi, C., & Beyeler, E. (2019). Neurobiological links between stress and anxiety. Neurobiology of Stress, 11(100191), 1-9. https://doi.org/10.1016/j.ynstr.2019.100191

39 Davis, A. E., Nathanson, J., Attwood. K., Sinha, A. A., Seiffert-Sinha, K. (2024). A retrospective analysis of patient-reported physical and psychological stressors as trigger factors in autoimmune bullous disease. Archives of Dermatological Research, 316(515), 1-4. https://doi.org/10.1007/s00403-024-03240-5

40 Paat, Y., Hope, T. L., Ferreira-Pinto, J. B., & Alvarez, H. O. (2024). A bio-psycho-social approach to understanding optimism and pessimism in response to stress. European Journal of Investigation in Health, Psychology and Education, 14, 2671-2685. https://doi.org/10.3390/ejihpe14100176

41 Selye, H. (1936). A syndrome produced by diverse nocuous agents. Nature, 138, 32. DOI: 10.1038/138032a0

42 Selye, H. (1936). A syndrome produced by diverse nocuous agents. Nature, 138, 32. DOI: 10.1038/138032a0

43 Selye, H. (1936). A syndrome produced by diverse nocuous agents. Nature, 138, 32. DOI: 10.1038/138032a0

44 Hechtman, L. (2012). Clinical naturopathic medicine. Elsevier Australia.

45 Daviu, N., Bruchas, M. R., Moghaddam, B., Sandi, C., & Beyeler, A. (2019). Neurobiological links between stress and anxiety. Neurobiology of Stress, 11(100191), 1-9. https://doi.org/10.1016/j.ynstr.2019.100191; Hechtman, L. (2012). Clinical Naturopathic

Medicine. Elsevier Australia.

46   Hechtman, L. (2012). *Clinical naturopathic medicine.* Elsevier Australia.

47   Hechtman, L. (2012). *Clinical naturopathic medicine.* Elsevier Australia.

48   Motzkin, J. C., Philippi, C. L., Wolf, R. C., Baskaya, M. K., & Koenigs, M. (2015). Ventromedial prefrontal cortex is critical for the regulation of amygdala activity in humans. *Biological Psychiatry, 77,* 276-284; Šimić, G., Tkalčić, M., Vukić, V., Mulc, D., Španić, E., Šagud, M., Olucha-Bordonou, F. E., Vukšić, M., & Hof, P. R. (2021). Understanding emotions: Origins and roles of the amygdala. *Biomolecules, 11*(6), 823. https://doi.org/10.3390/biom11060823

49   Giustino, T. F., & Maren, S. (2015). The role of the medial prefrontal cortex in the conditioning and extinction of fear. *Frontiers in Behavioural Neuroscience, 9*(298), 1-20. https://doi.org/10.3389/fnbeh.2015.00298; LeDoux, J. (1998). *The emotional brain.* Orion Books, Ltd.

50   LeDoux, J. (1998). *The emotional brain.* Orion Books, Ltd.

51   Hiser, J., & Koenigs, M. (2018). The multifaceted role of the ventromedial prefrontal cortex in emotion, decision making, social cognition and psychopathology. *Biological Psychiatry, 83*(8), 638-647. https://doi.org/10.1016/j.biopsych.2017.10.030

52   Hiser, J., & Koenigs, M. (2018). The multifaceted role of the ventromedial prefrontal cortex in emotion, decision making, social cognition and psychopathology. *Biological Psychiatry, 83*(8), 638-647. https://doi.org/10.1016/j.biopsych.2017.10.030

53   LeDoux, J. (1998). *The emotional brain.* Orion Books, Ltd.

54   LeDoux, J. (1998). *The emotional brain.* Orion Books, Ltd.

55   LeDoux, J. (1998). *The emotional brain.* Orion Books, Ltd.

56   LeDoux, J. (1998). *The emotional brain.* Orion Books, Ltd.

57   Short, E., Ajjan, R., Barber, T. M., Benson, I., Higginbotham, V., Huckstepp, R., Kanamarlapudi, V., Mumwiro, N., Calimport, S. R.

G., & Bently, B. (2025). Adrenal cortex senescence: an age-related pathology? *Journal of Endocrinological Investigation, 48,*1-10. https://doi.org/10.1007/s40618-025-02566-9

58 Short, E., Ajjan, R., Barber, T. M., Benson, I., Higginbotham, V., Huckstepp, R., Kanamarlapudi, V., Mumwiro, N., Calimport, S. R. G., & Bently, B. (2025). Adrenal cortex senescence: an age-related pathology? *Journal of Endocrinological Investigation, 48,*1-10. https://doi.org/10.1007/s40618-025-02566-9

59 LeDoux, J. (1998). *The emotional brain.* Orion Books, Ltd.

60 LeDoux, J. (1998). *The emotional brain.* Orion Books, Ltd.

61 Sherwood, L. (2001). *Human physiology: From cells to systems.* (4th ed.). Brooks/Cole.

62 Sherwood, L. (2001). *Human physiology: From cells to systems.* (4th ed.). Brooks/Cole.

63 Sherwood, L. (2001). *Human physiology: From cells to systems.* (4th ed.). Brooks/Cole.

64 Goldstein, D. S. (2010). Adrenal responses to stress. *Cellular and Molecular Neurobiology, 30,* 1433-1440. https://doi.org/10.1007/s10571-010-9606-9

65 Selye, H. (1936). A syndrome produced by diverse nocuous agents. *Nature, 32.*

66 Selye, H. (1936). A syndrome produced by diverse nocuous agents. *Nature, 32.*

67 Selye, H. (1936). A syndrome produced by diverse nocuous agents. *Nature, 32.*

68 McCance, K. L., & Huether, S. E. (2019). *Pathophysiology: The biologic basis for disease in adults and children.* (8th ed.). Elsevier, Inc.

69 McCance, K. L., & Huether, S. E. (2019). *Pathophysiology: The biologic basis for disease in adults and children.* (8th ed.). Elsevier, Inc.

70 McCance, K. L., & Huether, S. E. (2019). *Pathophysiology:*

The biologic basis for disease in adults and children. (8th ed.). Elsevier, Inc.

71   Platt, M. E. (2014). *Adrenaline dominance: A revolutionary approach to wellness.* Clancy Lane Publishing.

72   Knezevic, E., Nenic, K., Milanovic, V., & Knezevic, N. N. (2023). The role of cortisol in chronic stress, neurodegenerative diseases, and psychological disorders. *Cells, 12*(23), 1-18. https://doi.org/10.3390/cells12232726; McCance, K. L., & Huether, S. E. (2019). *Pathophysiology: The biologic basis for disease in adults and children.* (8th ed.). Elsevier, Inc; Rohleder, N. (2019). Stress and inflammation – the need to address the gap in the transition between acute and chronic stress effects. *Psychoneuroendocrinology, 105,* 164-171. https://doi.org/10.1016/j.psyneuen.2019.02.021

73   Bauer, M. E., & Teixeira, A. L. (2019). Inflammation in psychiatric disorders: what comes first? *Annals from the New York Academy of Sciences, 1437*(1), 57-67. https://doi.org/10.1111/nyas.13712; Rohleder, N. (2019). Stress and inflammation – the need to address the gap in the transition between acute and chronic stress effects. *Psychoneuroendocrinology, 105,* 164-171. https://doi.org/10.1016/j.psyneuen.2019.02.021

74   Katrinli, S., Oliveira, N. C. S., Felger, J. C., Michopoulos, V., & Smith, A. K. (2022). The role of the immune system in posttraumatic stress disorder. *Translation Psychiatry, 12*(313), 1-14. https://doi.org/10.1038/s41398-022-02094-7; Michopoulos, V., Powers, A., Gillespie, C. F., Ressler, K.J., & Jovanovic, T. (2017). Inflammation in fear- and anxiety-based disorders: PTSD, GAD, and beyond. *Neuropsychopharmacology Reviews, 42,* 254-270. https://doi.org/10.1038/npp.2016.146;

75   Knezevic, E., Nenic, K., Milanovic, V., & Knezevic, N. N. (2023). The role of cortisol in chronic stress, neurodegenerative diseases, and psychological disorders. *Cells, 12*(23), Article 2726. DOI: https://doi.org/10.3390/cells12232726; Wilcox, N. S., Amit, U.,

Reibel, J. B., Berlin, E., Howell, K., & Ky, B. (2024). Cardiovascular disease and cancer: shared risk factors and mechanisms. *Nature Reviews Cardiology, 21*(9), 617-631. https://doi.org/10.1038/s41569-024-01017-x; Yu, X., Pu, H., Voss, M. (2024). Overview of anti-inflammatory diets and their promising effects on non-communicable diseases. *British Journal of Nutrition, 132*(7), 898-918. https://doi.org/10.1017/S0007114524001405

76 McCance, K. L., & Huether, S. E. (2019). *Pathophysiology: The biologic basis for disease in adults and children.* (8th ed.). Elsevier, Inc.

77 Hechtman, L. (2012). *Clinical naturopathic medicine.* Elsevier Australia.

78 Hechtman, L. (2012). *Clinical naturopathic medicine.* Elsevier Australia.

79 Hechtman, L. (2012). *Clinical naturopathic medicine.* Elsevier Australia.

80 Hechtman, L. (2012). *Clinical naturopathic medicine.* Elsevier Australia.

81 Hechtman, L. (2012). *Clinical naturopathic medicine.* Elsevier Australia.

82 Guidi, J., Lucente, M., Sonino, N., & Fava, G. A. (2021). Allostatic load and its impact on health: A systematic review. *Psychotherapy and Psychosomatics, 90*(1), 11-27. https://doi.org/10.1159/000510696

83 Hechtman, L. (2012). *Clinical naturopathic medicine.* Elsevier Australia.

84 Goldstein, D. S. (2010). Adrenal responses to stress. *Cellular and Molecular Neurobiology, 30,* 1433-1440. https://doi.org/10.1007/s10571-010-9606-9

85 Rohleder, N. (2019). Stress and inflammation – the need to address the gap in the transition between acute and chronic stress effects. *Psychoneuroendocrinology, 105,* 164-171. https://doi.

org/10.1016/j.psyneuen.2019.02.021

86 Toufexis, D., Rivarola, M. A., Lara, H., & Viau, V. (2014). Stress and the reproductive axis. *Journal of Neuroendocrinology, 26*(9), 573-586. https://doi.org/10.1111/jne.12179

87 Odetayo, A. F., Akhigbe, R. E., Bassey, G. E., Hamed, M. A., & Olayaki, L. A. (2024). Impact of stress on male fertility: role of gonadotropin inhibitory hormone. *Frontiers in Endocrinology, 14*(1329564), 1-11. https://doi.org/10.3389/fendo.2023.1329564; Toufexis, D., Rivarola, M. A., Lara, H., & Viau, V. (2014). Stress and the reproductive axis. *Journal of Neuroendocrinology, 26*(9), 573-586. https://doi.org/10.1111/jne.12179

88 Zhu, Y., Wu, X., Zhou, R., Sie, O., Niu, Z., Wang, F., & Fang, Y. (2020). Hypothalamic-pituitary-end-organ axes: Hormone function in female patients with major depressive disorder. *Neuroscience Bulletin, 37*(8), 1176-1187. https://doi.org/10.1007/s12264-021-00689-6

89 Fischer, S., Strahler, J., Markert, C., Skoluda, N., Doerr, J. M., Kappert, M., & Nater, U. M. (2019). Effects of acute stress on the hypothalamic-pituitary-thyroid (HPT) axis. Psychoneuroimmunology, 107(S), 1-81. https://doi.org/10.1016/j.psyneuen.2019.104438; Odetayo, A. F., Akhigbe, R. E., Bassey, G. E., Hamed, M. A., & Olayaki, L. A. (2024). Impact of stress on male fertility: role of gonadotropin inhibitory hormone. *Frontiers in Endocrinology, 14*(1329564), 1-11. https://doi.org/10.3389/fendo.2023.1329564

90 Davis, A. E., Nathanson, J., Attwood. K., Sinha, A. A., Seiffert-Sinha, K. (2024). A retrospective analysis of patient-reported physical and psychological stressors as trigger factors in autoimmune bullous disease. *Archives of Dermatological Research, 316*(515), 1-4. https://doi.org/10.1007/s00403-024-03240-5

91 Iwaszczuk, P., Loziac, W., Szczeklik, W., & Musialek, P. (2021). Patient periprocedural stress in cardiovascular medicine: Friend or foe? *Advances in Interventional Cardiology, 17, 3*(65), 259-

271. https://doi.org/10.5114/aic.2021.109176

92 Iwaszczuk, P., Loziac, W., Szczeklik, W., & Musialek, P. (2021). Patient periprocedural stress in cardiovascular medicine: Friend or foe? *Advances in Interventional Cardiology, 17, 3*(65), 259-271. https://doi.org/10.5114/aic.2021.109176

93 Mosso-Vázquez, J. L., Gao, K., Wielderhold, B. K., & Wielderhold, M. D. (2014). Virtual reality for pain management in cardiac surgery. Cyberpsychology, Behaviour, and Social Networking, 17(6), 371-378. https://doi.org/10.1089/cyber.2014.0198

94 Ben-Ari, A., Benarroch, F., Sela, Y., & Margalit, D. (2020). Risk factors for the development of medical stress syndrome following surgical intervention. *Journal of Paediatric Surgery, 55,*(9) 1685-1690. https://doi.org/10.1016/j.jpedsurg.2019.11.011

95 Ben-Ari, A., Benarroch, F., Sela, Y., & Margalit, D. (2020). Risk factors for the development of medical stress syndrome following surgical intervention. *Journal of Paediatric Surgery, 55,*(9) 1685-1690. https://doi.org/10.1016/j.jpedsurg.2019.11.011

96 Lim, A. G., & McKenzie, G. (2006). *Australia New Zealand Nursing Drug Handbook.* Lippincott Williams and Wilkins.

97 Papatriantafyllou, E., Efthymiou, D., Markopoulou, M., Sakellariou, E., & Vassilopoulou, E. (2022). The effects of use of long-term second-generation antipsychotics on liver and kidney function: A prospective study. *Diseases, 10*(48), 1-10. https://doi.org/10.3390/diseases10030048

98 Atici, S., Cinel, I., Cinel, L., Doruk, N., Eskandari, G., & Oral, U. (2005). Liver and kidney toxicity in chronic use of opioids: An experimental long term treatment model. *Journal of Biosciences, 30,* 245-252. https://doi.org/10.1007/BF02703705

99 Atici, S., Cinel, I., Cinel, L., Doruk, N., Eskandari, G., & Oral, U. (2005). Liver and kidney toxicity in chronic use of opioids: An experimental long term treatment model. *Journal of Biosciences, 30,* 245-252. https://doi.org/10.1007/BF02703705

100   Nehlsen-Cannarlla, S. L. (1998). Cellular responses to moderate and heavy exercise. *Canadian Journal of Physiology and Pharmacology, 76*(5), 485-489. https://doi.org/10.1139/cjpp-76-5-485

101   Taylor, R. R., & Halliday, E. J. (1965). Beta-adrenergic blockade in the treatment of exercise-induced paroxysmal ventricular tachycardia. *Circulation, 32*(5), 778-781. https://doi.org/10.1161/01.CIR.32.5.778

102   Damiot, A., Pinto, A. J., Turner, J. E., & Gualano, B. (2020). Immunological implications of physical inactivity among older adults during the COVID-19 pandemic. Gerontology, 66(5),1-8. https://doi.org/10.1159/000509216

103   McCauley, M., Zafar, S., & van den Broek, N. (2020). Maternal multi-morbidity during pregnancy and after childbirth in women in low- and middle-income countries: A systematic literature review. *BMC Pregnancy and Childbirth, 20*(637), 1-10. https://doi.org/10.1186/s12884-020-03303-1

104   McNab, S., Fisher, J., Honikman, S., Muvhu, L., Levine, R., Chorwe-Sungani, G., Bar-Zeev, S., Degefie Hailegebriel, T., Yusuf, I., Chowdhary, N., Rahman, A., Bolton, P., Mershon, C., Bormet, M., Henry-Ernest, D., Portela, A., Stalls, S. (2022). Comment: silent burden no more: a global call to action to prioritize perinatal mental health. *BMC Pregnancy and Childbirth, 22*(308), 1-4. https://doi.org/10.1186/s12884-022-04645-8

105   McCauley, M., Zafar, S., & van den Broek, N. (2020). Maternal multi-morbidity during pregnancy and after childbirth in women in low- and middle-income countries: A systematic literature review. *BMC Pregnancy and Childbirth, 20*(637), 1-10. https://doi.org/10.1186/s12884-020-03303-1

106   Morgan, J., Bauer, S., Whitsel, A., & Combs, C. A. (2022). Society for maternal-fetal medicine special statement: Postpartum visit checklists for normal pregnancy and complicated pregnancy. *American Journal of Obstetrics and Gynaecology, 227*(4),

B2-B8. https://doi.org/10.1016/j.ajog.2022.06.007

107   Incollingo Rodriguez, A. C., Dunkel Schetter, C., Brewis, A., & Tomiyama, A. J. (2019). The psychological burden of baby weight: Pregnancy, weight stigma and maternal health. *Social Science & Medicine, 235*(112401), 1-10. https://doi.org/10.1016/j.socscimed.2019.112401

108   Incollingo Rodriguez, A. C., Dunkel Schetter, C., Brewis, A., & Tomiyama, A. J. (2019). The psychological burden of baby weight: Pregnancy, weight stigma and maternal health. *Social Science & Medicine, 235*(112401), 1-10. https://doi.org/10.1016/j.socscimed.2019.112401

109   Incollingo Rodriguez, A. C., Dunkel Schetter, C., Brewis, A., & Tomiyama, A. J. (2019). The psychological burden of baby weight: Pregnancy, weight stigma and maternal health. *Social Science & Medicine, 235*(112401), 1-10. https://doi.org/10.1016/j.socscimed.2019.112401

110 Incollingo Rodriguez, A. C., Dunkel Schetter, C., Brewis, A., & Tomiyama, A. J. (2019). The psychological burden of baby weight: Pregnancy, weight stigma and maternal health. *Social Science & Medicine, 235*(112401), 1-10. https://doi.org/10.1016/j.socscimed.2019.112401

111 World Health Organisation. (2023, July 27). *Ionizing radiation and health effects.* Ionizing radiation and health effects

112 World Health Organisation. (2020, October 26). *Radiation: Ionizing radiation.* Radiation: Ionizing radiation

113 World Health Organisation. (2020, October 26). *Radiation: Ionizing radiation.* Radiation: Ionizing radiation

114 World Health Organisation. (2020, October 26). *Radiation: Ionizing radiation.* Radiation: Ionizing radiation

115 AbuAlRoos, N. J., Amin, N. A B., & Zainon, R. (2019). Conventional and new lead-free radiation shielding materials for radiation protection in nuclear medicine: A review. *Radiation*

Physics and Chemistry, 165(108439). https://doi.org/10.1016/j.radphyschem.2019.108439

116 World Health Organisation. (2020, October 26). *Radiation: Ionizing radiation.* Radiation: Ionizing radiation

117 World Health Organisation. (2020, October 26). *Radiation: Ionizing radiation.* Radiation: Ionizing radiation

118 World Health Organisation. (2020, October 26). *Radiation: Ionizing radiation.* Radiation: Ionizing radiation

119 World Health Organisation. (2020, October 26). *Radiation: Ionizing radiation.* Radiation: Ionizing radiation

120 World Health Organisation. (2023, July 27). *Ionizing radiation and health effects.* Ionizing radiation and health effects

121 Bardelčíková, A., Šoltys, J., Mojžiš, J. (2023). Oxidative stress, inflammation and colorectal cancer: An overview. *Antioxidants, 12*(901), 1-17. https://doi.org/10.3390/antiox12040901

122 World Health Organisation. (2023, July 27). *Ionizing radiation and health effects.* Ionizing radiation and health effects

123 World Health Organisation. (2023, July 27). *Ionizing radiation and health effects.* Ionizing radiation and health effects

124 Zhang, Y., Gao, Y., Liu, Q. S., Zhou, Q., & Jiang, G. (2024). Chemical contaminants in blood and their implications in chronic diseases. *Journal of Hazardous Materials, 466*(133511), 1-15. https://doi.org/10.1016/j.jhazmat.2024.133511

125 Zhang, Y., Gao, Y., Liu, Q. S., Zhou, Q., & Jiang, G. (2024). Chemical contaminants in blood and their implications in chronic diseases. *Journal of Hazardous Materials, 466*(133511), 1-15. https://doi.org/10.1016/j.jhazmat.2024.133511

126 Zhang, Y., Gao, Y., Liu, Q. S., Zhou, Q., & Jiang, G. (2024). Chemical contaminants in blood and their implications in chronic diseases. *Journal of Hazardous Materials, 466*(133511), 1-15. https://doi.org/10.1016/j.jhazmat.2024.133511

127 Zhang, Y., Gao, Y., Liu, Q. S., Zhou, Q., & Jiang,

G. (2024). Chemical contaminants in blood and their implications in chronic diseases. *Journal of Hazardous Materials, 466*(133511), 1-15. https://doi.org/10.1016/j.jhazmat.2024.133511

128   Kumar, M., Kumar Sarma, D., Shubham, S., Kumawat, M., Verma, V., Prakash, A., & Tiwari, R. (2020). Environmental endocrine-disrupting chemical exposure: Role in non-communicable diseases. *Frontiers in Public Health, 8*(553850), 1-28. https://doi.org/10.3389/fpubh.2020.553850; Zhang, Y., Gao, Y., Liu, Q. S., Zhou, Q., & Jiang, G. (2024). Chemical contaminants in blood and their implications in chronic diseases. *Journal of Hazardous Materials, 466*(133511), 1-15. https://doi.org/10.1016/j.jhazmat.2024.133511

129   Kumar, M., Kumar Sarma, D., Shubham, S., Kumawat, M., Verma, V., Prakash, A., & Tiwari, R. (2020). Environmental endocrine-disrupting chemical exposure: Role in non-communicable diseases. *Frontiers in Public Health, 8*(553850), 1-28. https://doi.org/10.3389/fpubh.2020.553850

130   Kumar, M., Kumar Sarma, D., Shubham, S., Kumawat, M., Verma, V., Prakash, A., & Tiwari, R. (2020). Environmental endocrine-disrupting chemical exposure: Role in non-communicable diseases. *Frontiers in Public Health, 8*(553850), 1-28. https://doi.org/10.3389/fpubh.2020.553850

131   Manzoor, M. F., Tariq, T., Fatima, B., Sahar, A., Tariq, F., Munir, S., Khan, S., Ranjha, M. M. A. N., Sameen, A., Zeng, X., & Ibrahim, S. A. (2022). An insight into bisphenol A, food exposure and its adverse effects on health: A review. *Frontiers in Nutrition, (9)*1047827, 1-16. https://doi.org/10.3389/fnut.2022.1047827

132   Manzoor, M. F., Tariq, T., Fatima, B., Sahar, A., Tariq, F., Munir, S., Khan, S., Ranjha, M. M. A. N., Sameen, A., Zeng, X., & Ibrahim, S. A. (2022). An insight into bisphenol A, food exposure and its adverse effects on health: A review.

*Frontiers in Nutrition, (9)*1047827, 1-16. https://doi.org/10.3389/fnut.2022.1047827

133   Kumar, M., Kumar Sarma, D., Shubham, S., Kumawat, M., Verma, V., Prakash, A., & Tiwari, R. (2020). Environmental endocrine-disrupting chemical exposure: Role in non-communicable diseases. *Frontiers in Public Health, 8*(553850), 1-28. https://doi.org/10.3389/fpubh.2020.553850

134   Arias-Pérez, R. D., Taborda, N. A., Gómez, D. M., Narvaez, J. F., Porras, J., & Hernandez, J. C. (2020). Inflammatory effects of particulate matter air pollution. *Environmental Science and Pollution Research, 27,* 42390–42404. https://doi.org/10.1007/s11356-020-10574-w

135   Arias-Pérez, R. D., Taborda, N. A., Gómez, D. M., Narvaez, J. F., Porras, J., & Hernandez, J. C. (2020). Inflammatory effects of particulate matter air pollution. *Environmental Science and Pollution Research, 27,* 42390–42404. https://doi.org/10.1007/s11356-020-10574-w

136   Arias-Pérez, R. D., Taborda, N. A., Gómez, D. M., Narvaez, J. F., Porras, J., & Hernandez, J. C. (2020). Inflammatory effects of particulate matter air pollution. *Environmental Science and Pollution Research, 27,* 42390–42404. https://doi.org/10.1007/s11356-020-10574-w

137   Angon, P. B., Islam, M. S., KC, S., Das, A., Anjum, N., Poudel, A., & Suchi, S. A. (2024). Sources, effects and present perspectives of heavy metals contamination: Soil, plants and human food chain. *Heliyon, 10*(e28357), 1-15. https://doi.org/10.1016/j.heliyon.2024.e28357

138   Angon, P. B., Islam, M. S., KC, S., Das, A., Anjum, N., Poudel, A., & Suchi, S. A. (2024). Sources, effects and present perspectives of heavy metals contamination: Soil, plants and human food chain. *Heliyon, 10*(e28357), 1-15. https://doi.org/10.1016/j.heliyon.2024.e28357

139   Angon, P. B., Islam, M. S., KC, S., Das, A., Anjum, N., Poudel, A., & Suchi, S. A. (2024). Sources, effects and present perspectives of heavy metals contamination: Soil, plants and human food chain. *Heliyon, 10*(e28357), 1-15. https://doi.org/10.1016/j.heliyon.2024.e28357

140   Angon, P. B., Islam, M. S., KC, S., Das, A., Anjum, N., Poudel, A., & Suchi, S. A. (2024). Sources, effects and present perspectives of heavy metals contamination: Soil, plants and human food chain. *Heliyon, 10*(e28357), 1-15. https://doi.org/10.1016/j.heliyon.2024.e28357

141   Litchtenstein, A. H., Appel, L. J., Vadiveloo, M., Hu, F. B., Kris-Etherton, P. M., Rebholz, C. M., Sacks, F. M., Thorndike, A. N., Van Horn, L., & Wylie-Rosett, J. (2021). 2021 Dietary guidance to improve cardiovascular health: A scientific statement from the American Heart Association. *Circulation, 144*, e472-e487. https://doi.org/10.1161/CIR.0000000000001031

142   Litchtenstein, A. H., Appel, L. J., Vadiveloo, M., Hu, F. B., Kris-Etherton, P. M., Rebholz, C. M., Sacks, F. M., Thorndike, A. N., Van Horn, L., & Wylie-Rosett, J. (2021). 2021 Dietary guidance to improve cardiovascular health: A scientific statement from the American Heart Association. *Circulation, 144*, e472-e487. https://doi.org/10.1161/CIR.0000000000001031

143   Litchtenstein, A. H., Appel, L. J., Vadiveloo, M., Hu, F. B., Kris-Etherton, P. M., Rebholz, C. M., Sacks, F. M., Thorndike, A. N., Van Horn, L., & Wylie-Rosett, J. (2021). 2021 Dietary guidance to improve cardiovascular health: A scientific statement from the American Heart Association. *Circulation, 144*, e472-e487. https://doi.org/10.1161/CIR.0000000000001031

144   Yu, X. P., Pu, H. M., Voss, M. (2024). Overview of anti-inflammatory diets and their promising effects on non-communicable diseases. *British Journal of Nutrition, 132*(7), 898-918. https://doi.org/10.1017/S0007114524001405

145   Di Giosia, P., Stamerra, C. A., Giorgini, P., Jamialahamdi, T., Butler, A. E., & Sahebkar, A. (2022). The role of nutrition in inflammaging. *Aging Research Reviews, 77*(101596), 1-11. https://doi.org/10.1016/j.arr.2022.101596

146   GBD 2021 Tobacco Forecasting Collaborators. (2024). Forecasting the effects of smoking prevalence scenarios on years of life lost and life expectancy from 2022 to 2050: A systematic analysis for the Global Burden of Disease Study 2021. *Lancet Public Health, 9*(10), e729-744.

147   Münzel, T., Hahad, O., Kuntic, M., Keaney Jr, J. F., Deanfield, J. E., & Daiber, A. (2020). Effects of tobacco cigarettes, e-cigarettes, and waterpipe smoking on endothelial function and clinical outcomes. *European Heart Journal, 41*, 4057-4070. https://doi.org/10.1093/eurheartj/ehaa460

148   Cohen, N., Fedewa, S., & Chen, A. Y. (2018). Epidemiology and demographics of head and neck cancer population. *Oral and Maxillofacial Surgery Clinics, 30*(4), 381-395. https://doi.org/10.1016/j.coms.2018.06.001; Münzel, T., Hahad, O., Kuntic, M., Keaney Jr, J. F., Deanfield, J. E., & Daiber, A. (2020). Effects of tobacco cigarettes, e-cigarettes, and waterpipe smoking on endothelial function and clinical outcomes. *European Heart Journal, 41*, 4057-4070. https://doi.org/10.1093/eurheartj/ehaa460

149   World Health Organisation. (2025). *Alcohol.* Alcohol

150   World Health Organisation. (2025). *Alcohol.* Alcohol

151   International Agency for Research on Cancer. (n.d.). *Agents classified by the IARC monographs, volumes 1-138 - IARC monographs on the identification of carcinogenic hazards to humans.* Agents Classified by the IARC Monographs, Volumes 1–138 – IARC Monographs on the Identification of Carcinogenic Hazards to Humans; World Health Organisation. (2023, January 4). *No level of alcohol consumption is safe for our health.* No level of alcohol consumption is safe for our health

152   World Health Organisation. (2023, January 4). *No level of alcohol consumption is safe for our health*. No level of alcohol consumption is safe for our health

153   Rehm, J., & Imtiaz, S. (2016). A narrative review of alcohol consumption as a risk factor for global burden of disease. *Substance Abuse Treatment, Prevention and Policy, 11*(37), 1-12. https://doi.org/10.1186/s13011-016-0081-2

154   Walinski, A., Sander, J., Gerlinger, G., Clemens, V., Meyer-Lindenberg, A., & Heinz, A. (2023). The effects of climate change on mental health. *Deutsches Arzteblatt International, 120,* 117-124. https://doi.org/10.3238/arztebl.m2022.0403

155   Walinski, A., Sander, J., Gerlinger, G., Clemens, V., Meyer-Lindenberg, A., & Heinz, A. (2023). The effects of climate change on mental health. *Deutsches Arzteblatt International, 120,* 117-124. https://doi.org/10.3238/arztebl.m2022.0403

156   deSouza, W.M., & Weaver, S. C. (2024). Effects of climate change and human activities on vector-borne diseases. *Nature Reviews Microbiology, 22,* 476-491. https://doi.org/10.1038/s41579-024-01026-0; Semenza, J. C., Rocklöv, J., & Ebi, K. L. (2022). Climate change and cascading risks from infectious disease. *Infectious Diseases and Therapy, 11,* 1371-1390. https://doi.org/10.1007/s40121-022-00647-3

157   Semenza, J. C., Rocklov, J., & Ebi, K. L. (2022). Climate change and cascading risks from infectious disease. *Infectious Diseases and Therapy, 11,* 1371-1390. https://doi.org/10.1007/s40121-022-00647-3

158   Kaptchuck, T. J. (1947). *The Web That Has No Weaver: Understanding Chinese Medicine.* (2nd ed.). The McGraw-Hill Companies.

159   Kaptchuck, T. J. (1947). *The Web That Has No Weaver: Understanding Chinese Medicine.* (2nd ed.). The McGraw-Hill Companies.

160   Jamison, R. N., Anderson, K. O., & Slater, M. A. (1995). Weather changes and pain: Perceived influence of local climate on pain complaint in chronic pain patients. *Pain, 61*(2), 309-315. https://doi.org/10.1016/0304-3959(94)00215-Z

161   Jamison, R. N., Anderson, K. O., & Slater, M. A. (1995). Weather changes and pain: Perceived influence of local climate on pain complaint in chronic pain patients. *Pain, 61*(2), 309-315. https://doi.org/10.1016/0304-3959(94)00215-Z

162   Okunade, K. S. (2020). Human papillomavirus and cervical cancer. *Journal of Obstetrics and Gynaecology, 40*(5), 602-608. https://doi.org/10.1080/01443615.2019.1634030

163   Okunade, K. S. (2020). Human papilloma virus and cervical cancer. *Journal of Obstetrics and Gynaecology, 40*(5), 602-608. https://doi.org/10.1080/01443615.2019.1634030

164   Okunade, K. S. (2020). Human papilloma virus and cervical cancer. *Journal of Obstetrics and Gynaecology, 40*(5), 602-608. https://doi.org/10.1080/01443615.2019.1634030

165   Hsu, Y., Huang, D. Q., & Nguyen, M. H. (2023). Global burden of hepatitis B virus: Current status, missed opportunities and a call for action. *Nature Reviews Gastroenterology & Hepatology, 20*(8), 524-537. https://doi.org/10.1038/s41575-023-00760-9; Toh, M. R., Wong, E. Y. T., Wong, S. H., Ng, A. W. T., Loo, L., Chow, P. K., & Ngeow, J. (2023). Global epidemiology and genetics of hepatocellular carcinoma. *Gastroenterology, 164*(5), 766-782. https://doi.org/10.1053/j.gastro.2023.01.033; Wallace, M.C., Preen, D., Jeffrey, G. P., & Adams, L. A. (2015). The evolving epidemiology of hepatocellular carcinoma: a global perspective. *Expert Review of Gastroenterology and Hepatology, 9*(6), 765-779. https://doi-org.libraryproxy.griffith.edu.au/10.1586/17474124.2015.1028363

166   Toh, M. R., Wong, E. Y. T., Wong, S. H., Ng, A. W. T., Loo, L., Chow, P. K., & Ngeow, J. (2023). Global epidemiology

and genetics of hepatocellular carcinoma. *Gastroenterology, 164*(5), 766-782. https://doi.org/10.1053/j.gastro.2023.01.033

167   Hsu, Y., Huang, D. Q., & Nguyen, M. H. (2023). Global burden of hepatitis B virus: Current status, missed opportunities and a call for action. *Nature Reviews Gastroenterology & Hepatology, 20*(8), 524-537. https://doi.org/10.1038/s41575-023-00760-9; Lafaro, K. J., Demirjian, A. N., & Pawlik, T. M. (2015). Epidemiology of hepatocellular carcinoma. Surgical Oncology Clinics of North America, 24(1), 1-17. DOI: 10.1016/j.soc.2014.09.001

168   Querdasi, F. R., & Callaghan, B. L. (2023). A translational approach to the mind-brain-body connection. *Translational Issues in Psychological Science, 9*(2), 103-106. https://doi.org/10.1037/tps0000374

169   Querdasi, F. R., & Callaghan, B. L. (2023). A translational approach to the mind-brain-body connection. *Translational Issues in Psychological Science, 9*(2), 103-106. https://doi.org/10.1037/tps0000374

170   Querdasi, F. R., & Callaghan, B. L. (2023). A translational approach to the mind-brain-body connection. *Translational Issues in Psychological Science, 9*(2), 103-106. https://doi.org/10.1037/tps0000374

171   Denes, A., & Miyan, J. A. (2014). Brain-immune interactions in health and disease. *Frontiers in Neuroscience, 8*(382), 1-2. https://doi.org/10.3389/fnins.2014.00382

172   Maier, S. F. (2003). Bi-directional immune-brain communication: Implications for understanding stress, pain, and cognition. *Brain, Behaviour, and Immunity, 17*(2), 69-85. https://doi.org/10.1016/S0889-1591(03)00032-1

173   Maier, S. F. (2003). Bi-directional immune-brain communication: Implications for understanding stress, pain, and cognition. *Brain, Behaviour, and Immunity, 17*(2), 69-85. https://doi.org/10.1016/S0889-1591(03)00032-1

174   Johnson, C. E., & Naik, H. B. (2025). Microbiome perturbations in hidradenitis suppurativa. *Dermatologic Clinics, 43*,(2) 193-202. https://doi.org/10.1016/j.det.2024.12.005

175   Johnson, C. E., & Naik, H. B. (2025). Microbiome perturbations in hidradenitis suppurativa. *Dermatologic Clinics, 43*,(2) 193-202. https://doi.org/10.1016/j.det.2024.12.005; Peirce, J. M., & Alviña, K. (2019). The role of inflammation and the gut microbiome in depression and anxiety. *Journal of Neuroscience Research, 97,* 1223-1241. https://doi.org/10.1002/jnr.24476

176   Peirce, J. M., & Alviña, K. (2019). The role of inflammation and the gut microbiome in depression and anxiety. *Journal of Neuroscience Research, 97,* 1223-1241. https://doi.org/10.1002/jnr.24476

177   Golshany, H., Helmy, S. A., Morsy, N. F. S., Kamal, A., Yu, Q., & Fan, L. (2025). The gut microbiome across the lifespan: How diet modulates our microbial ecosystem from infancy to the elderly. *International Journal of Food Sciences and Nutrition, 76*(2), 95-121. https://doi.org/10.1080/09637486.2024.2437472

178   Golshany, H., Helmy, S. A., Morsy, N. F. S., Kamal, A., Yu, Q., & Fan, L. (2025). The gut microbiome across the lifespan: How diet modulates our microbial ecosystem from infancy to the elderly. *International Journal of Food Sciences and Nutrition, 76*(2), 95-121. https://doi.org/10.1080/09637486.2024.2437472

179   Golshany, H., Helmy, S. A., Morsy, N. F. S., Kamal, A., Yu, Q., & Fan, L. (2025). The gut microbiome across the lifespan: How diet modulates our microbial ecosystem from infancy to the elderly. *International Journal of Food Sciences and Nutrition, 76*(2), 95-121. https://doi.org/10.1080/09637486.2024.2437472

180   Peirce, J. M., & Alviña, K. (2019). The role of inflammation and the gut microbiome in depression and anxiety. *Journal of Neuroscience Research, 97,* 1223-1241. https://doi.org/10.1002/jnr.24476

181   Peirce, J. M., & Alviña, K. (2019). The role of inflammation and the gut microbiome in depression and anxiety. *Journal of Neuroscience Research, 97,* 1223-1241. https://doi. org/10.1002/jnr.24476

182   Peirce, J. M., & Alviña, K. (2019). The role of inflammation and the gut microbiome in depression and anxiety. *Journal of Neuroscience Research, 97,* 1223-1241. https://doi. org/10.1002/jnr.24476

183   Peirce, J. M., & Alviña, K. (2019). The role of inflammation and the gut microbiome in depression and anxiety. *Journal of Neuroscience Research, 97,* 1223-1241. https://doi. org/10.1002/jnr.24476

184   Peirce, J. M., & Alviña, K. (2019). The role of inflammation and the gut microbiome in depression and anxiety. *Journal of Neuroscience Research, 97,* 1223-1241. https://doi. org/10.1002/jnr.24476

185   Peirce, J. M., & Alviña, K. (2019). The role of inflammation and the gut microbiome in depression and anxiety. *Journal of Neuroscience Research, 97,* 1223-1241. https://doi. org/10.1002/jnr.24476

186   Weng, M., Chiu, Y., Wei, P., Chiang, C., Fang, H., & Wei, S. (2019). Microbiota and gastrointestinal cancer. *Journal of Formosan Medical Association, 118,* S32-S41. https://doi. org/10.1016/j.jfma.2019.01.002

187   Weng, M., Chiu, Y., Wei, P., Chiang, C., Fang, H., & Wei, S. (2019). Microbiota and gastrointestinal cancer. *Journal of Formosan Medical Association, 118,* S32-S41. https://doi. org/10.1016/j.jfma.2019.01.002

188   Merriam-Webster,   Incorporated.   (n.d.). Psychosomatic. In *Merriam-Webster Dictionary.* Retrieved 2025, from *PSYCHOSOMATIC Definition & Meaning - Merriam-Webster*

189   Wolke, D., & Lereya, S. T. (2015). Long-term

effects of bullying. *Archives of Disease in Childhood, 100,*(9) 879-885. https://doi.org/10.1136/archdischild-2014-306667

190   Wolke, D., & Lereya, S. T. (2015). Long-term effects of bullying. *Archives of Disease in Childhood, 100,*(9) 879-885. https://doi.org/10.1136/archdischild-2014-306667

191   Wolke, D., & Lereya, S. T. (2015). Long-term effects of bullying. *Archives of Disease in Childhood, 100,*(9) 879-885. https://doi.org/10.1136/archdischild-2014-306667

192   Vanuytsel, T., Bercik, P., & Boeckxstaens, G. (2023). Understanding neuroimmune interactions in disorders of gut-brain interaction: from functional to immune-mediated disorders. *Gut, 72,*(4) 787-798. https://doi.org/10.1136/gutjnl-2020-320633

193   Vanuytsel, T., Bercik, P., & Boeckxstaens, G. (2023). Understanding neuroimmune interactions in disorders of gut-brain interaction: from functional to immune-mediated disorders. *Gut, 72,*(4) 787-798. https://doi.org/10.1136/gutjnl-2020-320633

194   Vanuytsel, T., Bercik, P., & Boeckxstaens, G. (2023). Understanding neuroimmune interactions in disorders of gut-brain interaction: from functional to immune-mediated disorders. *Gut, 72,*(4) 787-798. https://doi.org/10.1136/gutjnl-2020-320633

195   Hallett, M., Aybek, S., Dworetzky, B. A., McWhirter, L., Staab, J. P., & Stone, J. (2022). Functional neurological disorder: New subtypes and shared mechanisms. *The Lancet Neurology, 21,* 537-550. https://doi.org/10.1016/S1474-4422(21)00422-1

196   Demartini, B., Nisticò, V., Edwards, M. J., Gambini, O., & Priori, A. (2021). The pathophysiology of functional movement disorders. *Neuroscience and Biobehavioural Reviews, 120,* 387-400. https://doi.org/10.1016/j.neubiorev.2020.10.019

197   Demartini, B., Nisticò, V., Edwards, M. J., Gambini, O., & Priori, A. (2021). The pathophysiology of functional movement disorders. *Neuroscience and Biobehavioural Reviews, 120,* 387-400. https://doi.org/10.1016/j.neubiorev.2020.10.019

198   Demartini, B., Nisticò, V., Edwards, M. J., Gambini, O., & Priori, A. (2021). The pathophysiology of functional movement disorders. *Neuroscience and Biobehavioural Reviews, 120,* 387-400. https://doi.org/10.1016/j.neubiorev.2020.10.019

199   Demartini, B., Nisticò, V., Edwards, M. J., Gambini, O., & Priori, A. (2021). The pathophysiology of functional movement disorders. *Neuroscience and Biobehavioural Reviews, 120,* 387-400. https://doi.org/10.1016/j.neubiorev.2020.10.019

200   Guidi, J., Lucente, M., Sonino, N., & Fava, G. A. (2021). Allostatic load and its impact on health: A systematic review. *Psychotherapy and Psychosomatics, 90,*(1) 11-27. https://doi.org/10.1159/000510696

201   Guidi, J., Lucente, M., Sonino, N., & Fava, G. A. (2021). Allostatic load and its impact on health: A systematic review. *Psychotherapy and Psychosomatics, 90,*(1) 11-27. https://doi.org/10.1159/000510696

202   Guidi, J., Lucente, M., Sonino, N., & Fava, G. A. (2021). Allostatic load and its impact on health: A systematic review. *Psychotherapy and Psychosomatics, 90,*(1) 11-27. https://doi.org/10.1159/000510696

203   Myss, C., Shealy, C. N. (1988-1999). *The Creation of Health: The Emotional, Psychological, and Spiritual Responses That Promote Health and Healing.* Transworld Publishers.

204   Myss, C. (1996). *Anatomy of the Spirit: The Seven Stages of Power & Healing.* Transworld Publishers.

205   Christiansen, C. (2007). Adolf Meyer revisited: Connections between lifestyles, resilience and illness. *Journal of Occupational Science, 14*(2), https://doi.org/10.1080/14427591.2007.9686586

About The Author

Amy Lewis is a registered nurse with 15 years of experience in clinical practice. She began her education in health after finishing school on the Gold Coast, completing a Bachelor of Science at the University of Queensland in Brisbane with majors in biomedical science and neuroscience. In her third year, she received the Dean's Commendation for high achievement. Following her studies, she worked in the field of human anatomy for 18 years, spending many years performing cadaver dissections for teaching and learning at both the University of Queensland and Griffith University. Her dedication and skill were recognised in 2004 when she received the prestigious Royal College of Surgeons Dissection Prize.

In 2010, Amy completed a Bachelor of Nursing at Queensland University of Technology, followed by a Graduate Certificate in Acute Care Nursing in 2015. Since then, she has been teaching in the School of Nursing and Midwifery at Griffith University. She has also done extensive study in the field of complementary medicine, which includes completing a Diploma in Acupressure and Certificates in Clinical Aromatherapy, Holistic Herbal Therapy, and Hand Reflexology.

Amy is the author of *Motor and Sensory Pathways of the Nervous System: An Anatomical Atlas Guide*, in which she also completed all the illustrations within the book. She currently lives in Brisbane with her two rescue cats and enjoys time with family, long walks, art, and playing piano.

www.ingramcontent.com/pod-product-compliance
Lightning Source LLC
Chambersburg PA
CBHW070931280326
41934CB00009B/1832